MW01231771

the
Going Down
guide

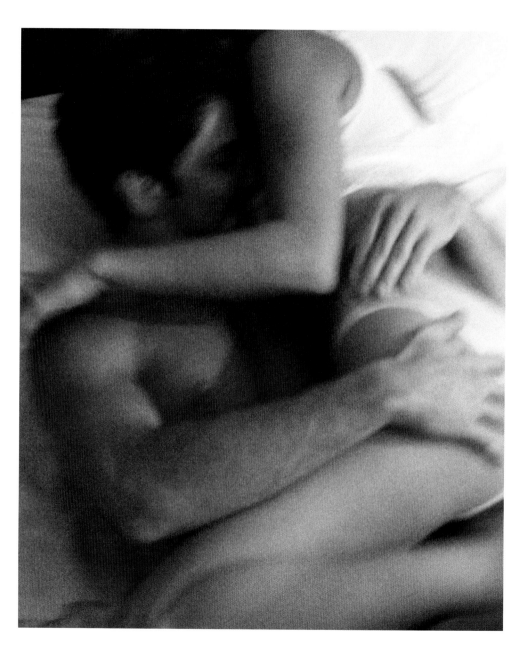

the
Going Down
guide

EMILY DUBBERLEY
AL NEEDHAM

St. Martin's Press ≋ New York

Copyright © 2009 Elwin Street Limited

All rights reserved. No part of this publication may be reproduced, stored in a
retrieval system, or transmitted in any form or by any means electronic, mechanical,
photocopying, recording, or otherwise without the prior written
permission of the copyright owner.

For information, address St. Martin's Press,
175 Fifth Avenue, New York, N.Y. 10010.

www.stmartins.com

Conceived and produced by
Elwin Street Productions
144 Liverpool Road
London N1 1LA
www.elwinstreet.com

Library of Congress Cataloging-in-Publication Data
Dubberley, Emily.
The going down guide : tongue tips and oral sex techniques for men and
women / Emily Dubberley. – 1st ed.
p. cm.
Includes index.
ISBN-13: 978-0-312-38474-6
ISBN-10: 0-312-38474-2
1. Oral sex. I. Title.
HQ31.5.O73D83 2009
613.9'6-dc22

First published in the United States by St Martin's Press

First U.S. Edition: 2009

10 9 8 7 6 5 4 3 2 1

Printed in Singapore

Contents

Introduction

When it comes to coming there's one act that's sure to hit the spot again and again: oral sex. Whether it's fantastic fellatio or consummate cunnilingus, by paying more than mere lip service to the act you're sure to put a smile on your lover's face.

As the name suggests, oral sex is about giving your lover pleasure with your lips, tongue, and sometimes (carefully!) teeth. Even when oral sex is bad, it's still quite good (assuming you've been careful with those teeth) but when it's good, it's better—and the difference between good oral and great oral is immense. While the former is all very nice, the latter can leave your lover trembling, incapable of speech, and grinning as if they've won the lottery on the same day that they've discovered the secret to eternal youth and been awarded the prize for "sexiest person on the planet." OK, maybe that's a slight exaggeration, but demonstrating your oral prowess will certainly make them come back for more again . . . and again . . . and again.

Physically, oral sex is great because it offers greater sensitivity than penetrative sex, allowing you to precisely target your lover's most intimate erogenous zones. Emotionally, it helps heighten the bond between you and your lover: if you've got your face buried in someone's bits, it suggests a certain closeness after all.

You might be sitting there reading this and feeling smug, certain that you know everything that there is to know about oral action. But there's one secret that every true oral connoisseur knows: no matter how skilled you are, there's always more to learn. Every man and woman is different: techniques that had your ex floating somewhere near the ceiling could leave a new lover doing a mental list of all the DIY that needs to be done around your home (or wishing you were doing it yourself). And techniques that made a previous partner push your head away from the meat of the matter and say "let's just kiss," could make another person writhe in glee.

Even if you're in a long term relationship, and both feel happy with your lot, there's still a good chance that you'll discover new ways to pleasure each other with a bit of experimentation. By varying your oral sex techniques, you can find new erogenous zones, figure out ways to last longer without your tongue or hand getting tired, and increase the intimacy between you and your lover.

It's pretty unlikely that your partner will object to a bit of oral experimentation. If they do, three little words should do the trick: "You come first." If you show that you're happy to spend hours lavishing your lover with oral attention then, chances are, it'll be easy to encourage them to return the favor.

So what are you waiting for? Get ready to (muff) dive in or show how deep (throat) your love is.

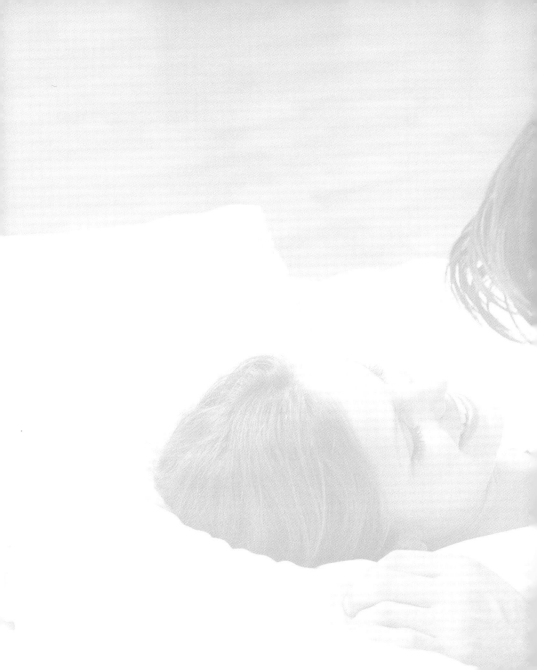

GETTING READY

All you need for a good oral sex session is a willing mouth and a
willing partner. However, with a bit of preparation, the
experience can be so much better for both of you.

1

First things first

Presentation matters, so to start with, make sure you've paid as much attention to your grooming ritual below the waist as above it.

Then there's the psychological side of things. Some people feel uncomfortable about giving or receiving oral sex. If your partner's one, a bit of encouragement may be required. While it's not acceptable to ask a partner to do anything that they don't enjoy, it is perfectly within your rights to insist on talking about why they're oral-phobic. If you're the one feeling uncomfortable at the idea, you should examine your own motivations. Oral sex is a hot addition to your sex life, whether giving or receiving, and it's a shame if you're so hung up about it that you don't get to experience it properly.

Assuming you've got all that lot out the way, it's down to the fun bit: warming your partner up. Although an unprompted oral session can be hot on occasion, spending time teasing your partner until every nerve is trembling is liable to lead to much more intense orgasms for them, and a much bigger ego boost for you. And once a lover is desperate for your touch? Don't just dive in there: remember your bedroom etiquette. You need to muff dive with manners or fellate with finesse. Politeness costs nothing, after all.

Are you ready? OK, we're going in . . .

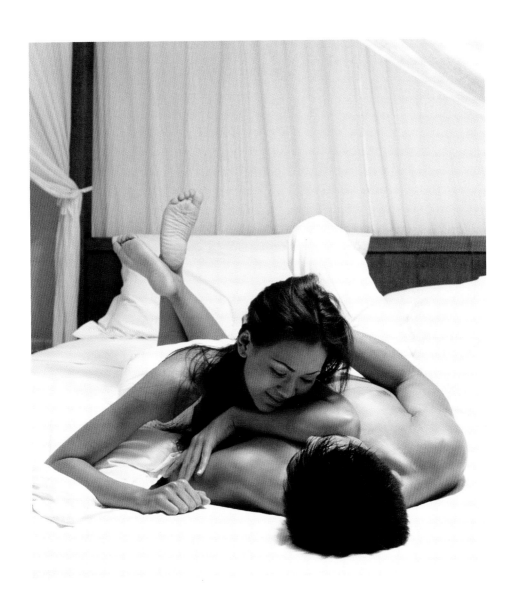

Sweet enough to eat

It may seem obvious but if you're in the mood for a hot oral session, you need to make sure that you're good enough to eat. You wouldn't eat off dirty dishes in a restaurant so you need to make sure that you offer a similarly well-polished pudenda or penis if you want your lover to dine on you. You don't need to be obsessive—vaginal deodorants are unnecessary and can upset the delicate balance down below. Similarly, over-frequent washing of the penis can cause irritation and lead to problems such as yeast infections or chafing. However, washing at least once per day, making sure to get into all the nooks and crannies (including under the foreskin and around the anus), will mean that you don't have anything unpleasant lurking to ruin "dinner."

If, despite having a good hygiene routine either you or your partner still smells unpleasant, take a trip to the STD clinic

TRY THIS NOW!

If your partner's hygiene leaves a little to be desired, try sharing a sexy shower or bath together before you get down to it. Comment on how great they smell and taste afterward. This will help resolve the issue without delivering a whopping blow to their ego, and is certainly far more effective than pointing out that they're a bit whiffy when they ask for oral.

together. Certain STDs change the way that your bits smell so it's worth ruling that option out.

Pheromones

Assuming that neither of you have STDs, but you still find the smell or taste unpleasant, there could be one other reason. People tend to be attracted to others who have a complementary immune system to their own. This is projected by the body through pheromones. When you meet someone that "smells right," you've got a good pheromonal match (either that or the fragrance they're wearing is well worth the money they spent on it). If you're less biologically compatible, you may find that you don't like the smell of your partner. While this doesn't mean you'll never be able to have a good relationship, it's certainly something you may want to consider if you're looking at long-term prospects. These pheromones are thought to be so powerful that a scientist in Boston has even set up a dating website that matches people by the way that they smell.

However, generally speaking, you should find that if you felt attracted to someone in the first place, there isn't a pheromonal problem. So just keep clean and drag your partner into the bath and you should be sorted.

Presentation matters

It's not just hygiene that's important. Presentation can make a difference too, and that's where pubes come in. These tricky little hairs take great pleasure in getting in the way, and getting one stuck in the back of the throat is an oral hazard. To avoid this, make sure that you comb through your pubes with your fingers before oral sex to get rid of any stragglers (it might be best to do this in the bathroom away from your partner rather than while they're in the room. It's not a sexy look). If you want to go a step further, pubic styling may be the way forward. Trimming makes a man's member look bigger and makes access to a woman's bits infinitely easier, so either way it's a winner.

Men have fairly limited options: basically, trimming it a bit or shaving it all off. Women, on the other hand, have a myriad of pubic styles to choose from. You can go for a Brazilian-style thin strip of hair on your pubic mound, or opt for having everything off in the Hollywood style. If you think diamonds are a girl's best friend then the Tiffany, in which you shape it into a square and dye it duck-egg blue, could be the shape for you; if you're more of a romantic, a classic heart could be your perfect style. Hell, you could even keep it simple and merely trim your bikini-line back neatly so that your lover's path is free of overhanging lady-garden. Don't feel obliged to get rid of your hair though: some men love the natural look. Just type "hairy women" into an Internet search engine and you'll see how popular they are.

If you do decide to go for some kind of hair removal, you may face itchy hair growing back. To avoid this, opt for waxing (take a painkiller an hour before you go in to help deaden the pain) or use a depilatory cream (making sure it's suitable for intimate areas first) as these tend to lead to less irritation than shaving.

If you prefer to shave, always use a new razor with a fresh blade. Make sure that you use lots of shaving cream so that the blade slides easily, and rinse it after every stroke with lukewarm water rather than hot water as this is less drying to the skin. Wash every last bit of shaving foam off carefully so that it doesn't cause irritation. Moisturize thoroughly with a lotion designed for sensitive skin and exfoliate gently using an exfoliating mitt or soft loofah for the first few days after you've shaved. This will help prevent irritating in-growing hairs when it starts to grow back.

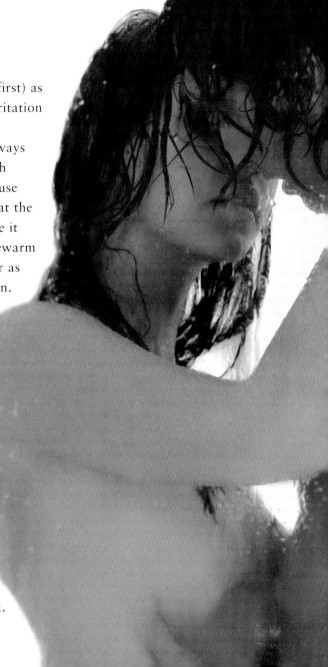

TIPS FOR HER FROM HIM
Pubic styling

The Brazilian

Otherwise known as the Landing Strip or the Badger, the Brazilian is sported by the type of woman who adores extensive oral attention—by subtly revealing as much skin on her pubic area as possible for full-on foreplay, while leaving just enough to remind her partner that she's very much an adult. It demonstrates she's willing to experiment, allowing her partner to explore nearly 80 percent more of her pubic area with licks, kisses and nibbles, without going to extreme lengths.

The Hollywood

The Hollywood signifies an extremely fastidious woman who's not afraid to experiment. She may be sacrificing base instincts for the sake of cleanliness (seeing as pubic hair traps natural scent, which is chock-full of natural pheromones, you're passing up a welter of chemical reactions), but is aware of the amazing sensations a bald lady-garden can provide. On the downside, she's not massively up for spontaneous sex when she gets a bit stubbly, and it's a look that demands constant time and attention.

The Tiffany

A natural high-maintenance show-off, the Tiffany girl seems to spend more time on presentation than performance. Yes, you have to admire the artistic interpretation, but you can't help wondering how much time she spent on it, and who helped. Plonking your nose into blue hair isn't the most naturally erotic thing in the world, to be honest, and the presence of a huge diamond right in front of your face sends out some terrifying subliminal messages to the more commitment-phobic male.

The Heart

See the Tiffany, but with creepier, Care Bear-related overtones. A very suitable look for redheads, though, with far less materialist overtones than the Tiffany. Best reserved for Valentines Day and anniversaries, really.

The Neat and Tidy

Probably the most satisfactory result for both parties, the Neat and Tidy woman goes for maximum sexiness with minimal effort. Most men like the comparative softness of lady-pubes, but are not so keen on feeling like they're having a smooch with their Geography teacher when they're down there. Not to mention the not-particularly-alluring appearance of spider-legs poking out of your underwear. Or the risk of getting one caught in your teeth.

Au naturel

Uncharitably described as "70s porno-bush," the Au naturel woman may be dismissed by certain men as someone not willing to put the effort in—but when you take into consideration the state of their own pubic topiary, they have little excuse to comment. When all's said and done, after all, what you do with your thatch is your own concern—we're just grateful to have access to it, at the end of the day . . .

Safety first

Just because you're perfectly groomed, don't assume that you're ready to go for it. Beauty is only skin deep and there could be something grim lurking below the surface. Yes, boring as it may sound, you also need to be aware of genital health issues before you get stuck in (or ask someone else to). Sexually transmitted diseases are on the increase and all manner of nasties from herpes to HIV can be passed on through oral sex.

While it's true to say that oral sex is a lower risk activity than vaginal or anal sex, that doesn't mean there's no risk. As such, make sure that you're careful. There have been cases of syphilis, gonorrhea, and HIV transmission through oral sex. Indeed, oral sex has been a major "driver" of the spread of syphilis in some areas.

And then there's herpes. To put it bluntly, if you or your lover has a cold sore (aka oral herpes) you shouldn't have oral sex. A herpes sore is fairly distinctive—just look up pictures on the Internet if you're not sure how to identify one, and if in doubt, refuse to let anyone with a spot on their lip go down on you. While it's not terminal, herpes is incurable and it's better to be safe than sorry. You should also be aware that the herpes virus can "shed" even when it's not visible which means it could be contagious even without an obvious spot. That doesn't mean that if you or a partner has herpes you should skip oral sex altogether but you should talk to your doctor about the risks and make sure that you're extra careful.

If you really want to be on the safe side during oral sex you can use a condom on men and a "latex dam" on women. This is a square of latex that can be used to cover the area being licked. If you can't find these dams at the drugstore, make your own from a flavoured condom. Simply cut the teat off then snip down the side. Voila! One square of latex that can be used to keep you safe. Don't try this with a normal condom as they taste revolting, particularly if they are coated with Nonoxynol-9 or spermicides.

It may seem like a pain but it's well worth a little bit of inconvenience to keep you safe and able to enjoy oral for years to come. Surely safe oral sex is better than no oral sex at all?

TRY THIS NOW!

Draw a non-reversible letter such as R or L on one side of the dam in non-toxic pen. As the dam has to be stretched over the genital region, it can 'ping' off. If that happens you'll be able to tell which way round the dam is supposed to go and you're not in danger of putting it back in position the wrong way round, with the side that's had genital contact against your tongue (and vice versa), which kind of defeats the object.

Fussy eater?

Once all the physical stuff is out of the way, it's time to move on to the psychological side of things. Like it or not, some people have hang-ups about oral sex, whether giving or receiving. They might feel that it's dirty or taboo (something that, conversely, can make it an extra turn-on for some people). They may feel insecure about their smell or taste, or feel squeamish about the idea of licking the genitals.

Women in particular may feel that it's wrong to abandon themselves sexually—the old "nice girls don't" stigma can kick in. If you're one of them, bear in mind that only 2.5 percent of men claim that giving oral doesn't turn them on at all, so that's 97.5 percent of men who get the horn from giving oral sex (and the other 2.5 percent clearly aren't worth dating). In fact, 55 percent of men list the taste of a woman as a top turn-on. You'll enjoy it even more if you're relaxed about it, explore each other's concerns and focus on the blissful intimacy that a good cunnilingus session entails. Some people feel uncomfortable about the idea of losing control and having an orgasm—or worse, peeing—while their partner is performing oral sex.

If you're the one who's insecure about receiving oral sex, and assuming you don't have any unresolved issues from previous bad experiences, relax. There's nothing wrong with the smell or taste of clean, healthy genitals. Taste yourself if you're so worried about it. See, it's really not that bad.

When it comes to urination, rest assured that you're safe. The body is designed to block the flow of urine during sexual arousal: just ask anyone who's into 'watersports' how tricky it is to break their body's conditioning (assuming, of course, that you know someone who'd admit the secrets of their kinky sex life to you. If not, there are plenty of online forums you can visit, if you really want to check this out).

As for feeling worried about coming, remind yourself that there's nothing wrong with letting go: that is the reason he's down there. As long as you feel comfortable with your partner and are happy to be sexual with him, it's simply giving him a reward for all his hard work. It won't give your partner power over you or make him love you any less. If anything, it will only increase the closeness between you. Don't be scared to share your concerns with your partner though: chances are, he'll be happy to reassure you. Oral sex is an intimate act and requires you to trust your partner—that's half the point (the other half

"When I was younger I used to hate it when a guy went down on me. It felt too personal and I didn't know where to look but closing my eyes felt rude. Then I met my current boyfriend, who absolutely loves giving me head. I was skeptical at first but he begged me so much that eventually I let him. It was one of the best decisions I ever made. Now I couldn't imagine our sex life without it."

LAURA, 28

being a damned good orgasm, of course). And the more relaxed you are, the quicker you're likely to reach climax.

Which brings us to a rather sticky subject: swallowing. Although women can get very wet and even ejaculate (of which more later), generally speaking, it's a lot more likely for a male orgasm to come complete with, well, come. The taste and sensation of swallowing semen isn't something that appeals to every woman's palate and this aversion could even lead a partner to decline administering oral sex at all.

If this is something that you're affected by, you may find it helpful to try some of the semen sweetening tricks in Chapter Three. However, if your partner balks at the very idea of swallowing, no matter how sweet it allegedly tastes, then you'll need to try harder if you want to win her round. You'll need to promise—and mean it—that you won't come in her mouth. Since this is one of the most common lies ever told, you may need to be particularly persuasive. And make sure you mean it! All it takes is one over-enthusiastic firing session and you'll be back to square one. While it can be all very lovely to come in a woman's mouth, if it stands between you and getting blow jobs at all, is it really that important? You can always come over her body or face instead, if that's something she doesn't object to. And if she does object? Are you honestly saying that it'll be the first time you've come into a handful of tissues? Get over it.

Unless you've had traumatic oral experiences, there's really no reason to worry about giving or receiving oral sex. Just relax, give it a go and you should be surprised at the results . . .

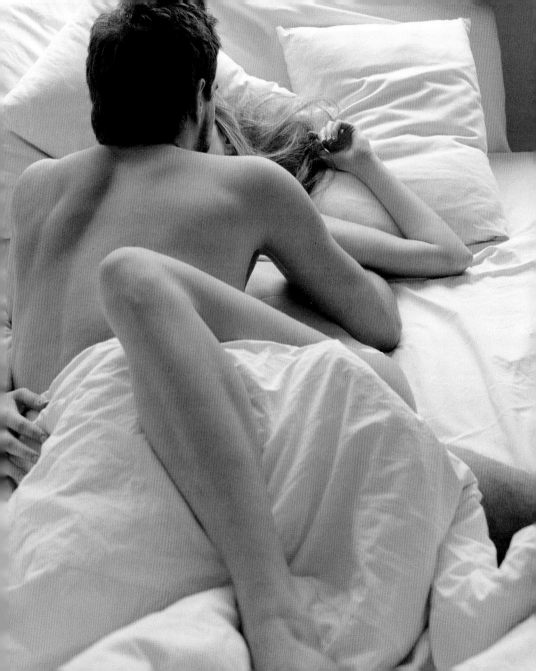

TIPS FOR HER FROM HIM
Common mistakes women make

1. *Giving up too early. Don't think that fellatio is a quick solution for getting us off the minute you clamp your lips around us. Pace yourself, take your time and don't panic if he's not automatically throwing ropes like Spider-Man—it doesn't mean you're no good at it, and neither does it mean he's not enjoying it.*

2. *Not mixing up techniques. There's more to fellatio than sucking, and the penis is far more complicated than women give credit for. You may be able to deep-throat a baguette, but if you're doing nothing but that, you'll find that oral familiarity breeds genital disinterest. Take time to discover what he likes to have done to different parts of his penis.*

3. *Not mixing up rhythms. Your lips, mouth and tongue can do a myriad of things your vagina can't. When you're down there, you're the one in control, and can dictate the pace at will, revving him up with enthusiastic mouth-bobbing one minute and then slithering your tongue down his shaft the next.*

4. *Forgetting about his balls. They like attention too. And I don't just mean oral attention—gently rubbing them or cupping them in your hand improves the sensations tenfold, and the slightest (and I mean slightest) pull on the bottom of his scrotum as he's about to come makes for an incredibly intense orgasm.*

5. Ignoring the rest of his body. We've got more than one erogenous zone, y'know, and we do like to be teased—so don't forget to put your hands on our ass to pull us into you, or brush your cheek along our inner thighs, or draw a line with your tongue from our bellybutton downward.

6. Doing too much, too soon. If you start bobbing your head like a heavy metal fan on crack, three things will happen; first, you'll get jaw-ache. Next, you'll look as if you're not enjoying it. Then he'll start thinking you don't want to do it, and feel guilty. Take your time.—spend time jerking him off while swizzling your tongue around the head of his penis.

7. Being too gentle. Our penis is designed to be able to take a lot more punishment than you think (and trust us, we've spent years testing our tolerance levels). While your bits require a little more gentleness, we can take a lot more punishment . . .

8. Using teeth. This is where we draw the line, in most cases. Unless we specifically ask for it, it's best to avoid dental contact; otherwise, we start to get a bit worried about having it bitten off.

9. Complaining that it's taking too long. Most women can't come from penetrative sex, but it doesn't mean their partners are lousy lays. Conversely, the fact that your man seems unable to climax from oral sex doesn't mean you're doing anything wrong. If you start pressuring him to come, he won't. Simple as that.

10. Grimacing when he ejaculates. It's not battery acid, you know.

Warming up

Now that all the boring stuff is out of the way, it's time for the fun to begin. Well, nearly. You wouldn't just get straight down to penetrative sex without any preamble (I hope) so why should oral sex be any different?

Get your partner eager for your lips and tongue. If they're already aroused and begging for your oral attentions before your tongue has even vaguely moved south, half the work will already be done. So spend time kissing your partner, demonstrating exactly how skilled your tongue is. Kiss your lover's neck, chest (yes, that works on lots of men too), and coccyx (the dimple at the base of the spine). And don't think you've got to be solely orally-fixated. Use your hands as well, and stroke your lover all over, caressing the side of the torso, the neck, the inner thighs, and the navel before moving onto more obvious erogenous zones.

If you're confident enough in your verbal seduction skills, whisper smutty suggestions into your lover's ear, or praise the way they look, smell, and taste. Say that you've been fantasising about going down on them and, ideally, mean it. The more enthusiastic you are about oral, the better it will be for both of you. Only move directly to the genitals once your lover is trembling and aching for your touch.

Bedroom etiquette

Once you get started, don't forget your manners. Although it can be tempting to just go for it, checking your partner's reaction as you go along is only polite. This is particularly important with a new lover, as you need to learn the blueprint to a whole new body. Don't be too hesitant in your attentions and don't just assume that what you're doing is bound to work because "it's worked on everyone else."

Check whether your partner wants you to use just your mouth or get hands involved too. Make sure you're not sucking too hard or too gently. Ask if you should move faster or slower, or even stay absolutely still so that they can move against you to a rhythm of their choosing. Ask these questions as you perform (well, during brief breaks—it's rude to speak with your mouth full), in a husky voice so that it doesn't feel like you're playing Twenty Questions. Alternatively, keep a close watch on your lover's body and it should show you what's hitting the spot.

Men sometimes release pre-come as they get closer to climax but that's not universal so don't rely on it as a signal. Similarly, some men will have a noticeably pulsing shaft immediately before climax, but that's by no means guaranteed. That said, if a man's penis does start to pulse it's a pretty safe bet that he's nearing the edge.

TIPS FOR HIM FROM HER
Common mistakes men make

1. *Attempting to beat the "World Tongue Speed Record." It is not a race. Speed is not essential and it certainly won't make her orgasm any quicker. Slow down and savor the flavor.*

2. *Going down without shaving first. Although there are some women out there who like it, generally it's a painful experience that makes it impossible to relax because you're too busy thinking about the chafing that you're going to be left with the next morning.*

3. *Relying on tongue alone to do the job. Yes, a tongue is a lovely thing on the genitals but it is possible for the fingers and tongue to move at the same time. Try it. She might like it.*

4. *Changing pace and technique every ten seconds so that the woman can't get into any sense of rhythm. The occasional teasing move away when a woman's close to coming is one thing: constantly doing it is quite another.*

5. *Being squeamish and licking so delicately, with such a look of disgust on your face, that the woman feels like you're performing oral as* community service. Women can tell when you're going down on them just to get the "favor" returned.

6. Similarly, looking up and saying "Is that enough yet?" If you're not going to at least pretend to enjoy it, don't bother.

7. Moving down to lick her anus without asking first. Some women like it but just as many feel squeamish—and if you move your tongue from anus to vagina, you can encourage yeast infections too. Not sexy. Save analingus for after you've talked about it with your partner.

8. Refusing to move when you're being pushed away after the woman's come, even when she's using all her strength. Yes, carrying on can sometimes lead to multiple orgasms but it can also be intensely painful.

9. Spitting on your partner's bits. OK, some women like the whole submissive kick but at least as many find it really offensive or hate the feeling of warm saliva dribbling over their bits. Check before you pull your porn moves out.

10. Biting. Unless you've been specifically asked to then just don't. Ever.

Signs of arousal

If your partner is aroused, you should find one or more of the following signals:

- ❀ Tensed muscles.
- ❀ A flushed chest or face.
- ❀ Increasingly engorged genitals.
- ❀ Hardening nipples (this varies from person to person).
- ❀ Gritted teeth (this can also indicate pain so make sure you haven't got a pubic hair caught between your teeth— while it's still attached to your lover).
- ❀ Heavy breathing.

Signs of boredom

Then there's spotting signs of boredom. If you notice any of the following, you may need to hone your technique:

- ❀ Changing the TV channel.
- ❀ Talking in complete sentences (particularly if they sound like something you'd hear in porn).
- ❀ Screaming "I'm coming, I'm coming, I'm coming," while their body stays completely relaxed.

Chances are, if you do something radically wrong, such as bite, your partner will tell you (or yelp in pain). Try not to respond defensively: it's bad enough that you've just inadvertently hurt your lover, without getting in a mood with them as well. And if your partner does something utterly wrong, don't just grin and bear it. Your partner will never understand what you really enjoy if you pretend that every single touch sends you into paroxysms.

As well as checking your partner is enjoying what you're doing, it's also important to check that they're relaxed. Not only will it make orgasm easier but if they're looking stressed, it could be because you're doing something wrong—or they're about to break wind and are trying to figure out the polite way to ask you to move.

Or course, there's no ideal way to deal with the above scenario: if sex was ideal there wouldn't be any breaking wind to face. However, there is one guaranteed way not to deal with it. Don't think that you can get it out and your partner won't notice. OK, confessing "You need to move, I'm going to fart," won't add romance to the equation but letting go is just as uncouth and has the added disadvantage of showing your partner zero respect. By far the best way to get out of the situation with your dignity intact and partner happy is to moan, "I need to kiss you," and drag them up toward you. After a few kisses, make your excuses to nip to the bathroom. Even better, fake a cramp and leap out of bed grasping your leg to "fix it." This gives you the perfect excuse to go to the bathroom as you "need to stretch your legs." OK, lying to a partner isn't cool but the odd white lie is forgivable.

Unpleasant bodily functions aside, there's only one more bit of essential etiquette: how to deal with the wet patch. First off, do your best to avoid it. Putting a towel down or agreeing not to spray your ejaculate around like an over-enthusiastic porn star are both good starts. They'll save you having to wash your sheets every night as well so it's an eco-friendly option as well. Should you get it on in such a passionate haze that you ignore the above advice and end up with a wet spot glaring you in the face, either agree to take it in turns to suffer wet-patch-sleeping, or better yet, try turning the sheets around as that should get the wet spot out of the "danger zone" and neither of you will end up lying in it. Then again, if you're the only one who's had oral sex administered, be fair and accept that the juices are your responsibility. Getting the orgasm and the dry patch just isn't fair.

By now, you should know everything that you need to have a perfectly acceptable oral session—but who wants one of those when there's the option of fabulous oral sex instead? Read on to discover how to give a brilliant blow job and consummate cunnilingus—and get ready to put a smile on your lover's face.

Dos and Don'ts

Do

1. Protect yourself against STDs.
2. Wash carefully beforehand.
3. Warm your lover up before going down (unless you're aiming for a fast and dirty oral quickie session).
4. Listen to your partner while you're going down on them, and always pay attention to their body language as much as their words.
5. Try to come quickly when you're receiving oral. No matter how much your partner loves administering it, they still want you to come before their tongue or jaw goes into spasm.

Don't

1. Give oral sex purely as a way to get it.
2. Break wind while your partner's down there.
3. Push your partner's head down when you fancy an oral session. Ask politely—or talk sexily and tease their body until they're in the mood.
4. Use your teeth.
5. Freak out about giving or receiving oral sex. It really can be a lot of fun. Honest.

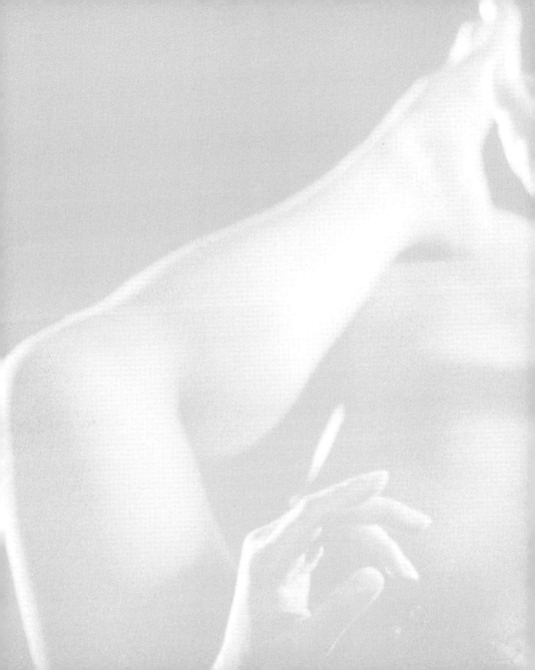

PLEASURING
A WOMAN

Oral sex is one of the easiest ways to give a woman an orgasm. As such, any man who's a cunnilingus king will be in demand—and the good news is that it's really not that complicated to be an oral expert with a technique she'll be raving about for years to come.

2

Look before you lick

You wouldn't eat a meal in the pitch dark, because you want
to know what you're eating, so why treat cunnilingus any
differently? A basic knowledge of female anatomy can make all
the difference and this is a tad trickier than it is with men.
Women's bits are hidden out of the way and vary hugely in
terms of size, shape, and sensitivity, whereas men tend to be a
lot more similar to each other. However, a little bit of
exploration should be all you need to refine your technique.
Look before you lap to learn what you're dealing with.

Spread your partner's legs and open up her labia (outer
lips)—or ask her to hold them open for you, if she's confident
enough. Now, enjoy the view. This is a very intimate act and
some women may feel unsettled so it's a good time to throw in
a few compliments. "You're so gorgeous," or "I love the way
you smell," will both go a long way in helping her chill out,
and relaxation is key for achieving great orgasms. By boosting
her confidence, you're decreasing your chances of ending up
with a cricked neck from being down there for hours.

Now you've got your partner beautifully open in front of
you, working from the outside in, you've got the labia majora,
or outer lips. These are the ones that are covered with pubes
(unless she's a shaven haven kind of girl, but you get the gist).
Lots of people ignore the outer lips when giving oral sex,
preferring to focus on the juicier inner lips, but the labia
majora are also sensitive to teasing, and can take a bit more
pressure than the clit and inner lips, so shouldn't be overlooked.

For example, use your fingers to hold open her outer lips and squeeze gently while your tongue gets to work on her clit and inner lips. Who said only women can multitask?

Now, look in between her lips. Toward the top, you'll see a nubbly bit covered by a tiny "hood" of skin (or prepuce). This is the clit. They come in all different shapes and sizes. Some are almost impossible to find, particularly in larger ladies with fatty pubic mounds, while others all but jump up and down shouting, "Lick me!"

If you have a hard time finding a clitoris, it doesn't mean that you're a rubbish lover. Some clits can be downright shy and retreat as far inside the hood as they can the second it looks like they're going to face anyone (or their tongue). If you encounter an elusive clit, ask your partner to show it to you. Not only will this show that you care about giving her pleasure but you'll also get a masturbation show—result! Once they've identified it, you should be able to keep track of it relatively easily. It's the bit that swells the most and feels the hardest

TRY THIS NOW!

Draw a picture of your partner's bits and ask her to put a cross on any areas she particularly likes licked, stroked, or nibbled. This is a good way to help even the shyest woman ask for what she wants. If she says she doesn't know, go down on her and help her put an X on the spot.

underneath your tongue—assuming you're teasing it in the right way, of course.

Moving down, you'll encounter the labia minora, or inner lips. These are packed with nerve endings that just love feeling a warm, wet tongue sliding over them. They also vary in size—some women worry that theirs hang down too low or are uneven, so again, reassurance is a good thing.

Then you have the vaginal opening. Some men make the mistake of assuming that's where all the action should go on, falsely believing that a tongue should just act as a miniature penis. While a good tongue-fucking can be very pleasurable, ignoring the clit and labia makes it a lot less likely that a woman will come. There are way more nerves in the clit than the vaginal opening so you're just making hard work for yourself.

Below the vaginal opening, you'll find the perineum—the area of skin between vagina and anus. Although some women are squeamish about any stimulation near the anus, this can also be sensitive, so try rubbing your tongue over it. Pleasuring every inch of her is far more likely to get the results that you want. Don't go for rimming (licking her anus) unless she asks you to though: perineal stimulation is wild enough to start with.

"I remember hearing some woman on a TV show say she couldn't understand how men can't find the clit because it's easy enough to remember: 'front and center.' I couldn't agree more!"

JEMMA, 32

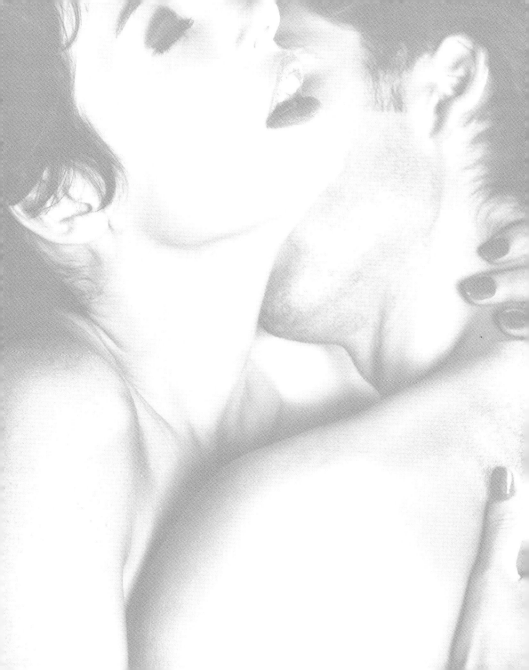

The cunnilingus commandments

There are some very basic rules to remember when going down on a woman that will enhance the experience for both of you.

Commandment One: Softly does it

Men tend to prefer more pressure than women do down below. As a result, a lot of guys wade in way too heavily during cunnilingus, following the "treat other people as you'd like to be treated" rule. This way lies chafing, pain, and getting your head pushed away (yeah, and you thought that was just because she was desperate for a good banging. Sorry to burst your bubble).

A cunnilingus king starts off incredibly gently. Imagine that you're licking a stamp made out of tissue paper that will rip if you apply too much pressure. Start by licking the clitoris through the hood—it can be too sensitive to touch directly before it gets fully aroused (and gets exceptionally sensitive after climax too, so back away from the clit once she's come). Run your tongue softly over her thighs, outer and inner labia, and around the entrance to her vagina. Build up a regular pattern, so she knows what's coming next. It makes it much easier for her to relax and aim toward climax.

Commandment Two: Shave

OK, there are one or two women out there who enjoy the sensation of stubble on their bits but they're in the distinct minority. No man can understand the pain of a sharp piece of stubble dragged over an erect clit (unless they have a penchant for masturbating using sandpaper), so unless you want to ruin the mood in the unsexiest way possible, shave before you go down. Please. Moisturizing is just an added bonus.

Commandment Three: Enjoy your meal

No woman's going to enjoy cunnilingus if you look bored, or worse, like you're doing it under duress. So make occasional eye contact with her, and tell her how great she looks, tastes, and feels. If you get hard when you're going down, tell your partner—it will make her even more likely to feel horny and come. Alternatively, blindfold her first so that she can't see how dull you find the entire thing. Then, as long as you don't audibly yawn, you should be OK.

TRY THIS NOW!

Start going down on your partner and work your way through each of the ten commandments (mentally—saying them out loud will so spoil the mood). Make a note of anything that makes a particularly big difference. And if your partner says that something really doesn't work for her, pay attention. Just because it's a commandment doesn't mean that it's more important than what your lover thinks. Sex manuals can only ever steer you in the right direction: your partner's the one who can tell you how to drive her crazy.

Commandment Four: Ask for it

Women often feel that men think cunnilingus is a chore. If you beg her to let you go down on her then she's much more likely to believe you really are into it. This will help her relax which will make it easier for her to come more quickly. So, it's a win/win situation: she gets off and you don't end up with a tired tongue.

Commandment Five: Use your lips…

All too many men think that oral sex involves flicking their tongue in and out snake-like, or worse, sticking their tongue out and then shaking their head from side to side. Porn has a lot to answer for. OK, the tongue is important, but don't underestimate what you can do with your lips. The inside of the lips is exceptionally soft, and can feel incredible rubbed gently over the tip of the clit. Or try capturing the clit between your lips and gently sucking on it (don't go for the full-on hoover approach unless you've been told that this is exactly what she wants. Again, less is more). Even kissing the clit can provoke a steamy reaction. So press your lips to hers, and enjoy the most intimate possible kiss.

Commandment Six: And your tongue…

However, the tongue is all-important in great oral. Again, use the underside as well as the top of the tongue as both give a different sensation. If you have a hard time holding back your ministrations (see Softly does it), using the underside of your tongue will limit the amount of pressure that you can apply.

Vary the types of strokes you use, from lapping to flicking to simply keeping your tongue pressed against her while she moves her body against your face. Try moving up and down, and from side to side, paying attention to the way that she responds. And when you find something she likes, keep at it. Unless, of course, you feel like being a teasing swine (or want her to hit you).

Commandment Seven: But not teeth

Biting is something that's best kept strictly away from the genitals. Yes, there are some people who get off on pain but they'll tell you, with any luck. So, unless you've been asked explicitly, keep your teeth well covered. Extremely gentle nibbling is the only exception but what feels soft to you may well feel like you're trying to bite off her clit to her, so it's best left until you know someone's bodily reactions well enough to gauge exactly how she's feeling about every nip.

Commandment Eight: A finger of fun

A lot of men treat oral sex and fingering as entirely different things, but combining the two means that you can deliver the double whammy of clitoral and vaginal/G-spot stimulation. And if you can keep your finger and tongue to the same rhythm then you're likely to elicit a screamingly good response.

Commandment Nine: A change isn't as good as a rest

You're getting down and dirty, glad that you spent your youth practicing tongue-twisters and she's writhing and clearly loving every second of it. Do you a) carry on with what you're doing, making a mental note to do it again in the future, or b) change to something entirely different. The answer should be obvious but you'd be amazed at how many men go for changing the pace just as they're about to hit the jackpot. So, if you're doing

---

"When a guy's going down on me I always worry that he's bored. It probably wasn't helped by the guy who got down there and after 30 seconds looked up at me and said "Is that enough yet?" The answer was an emphatic yes—it was such a turn off thinking he was down there counting the seconds until he could have sex with me and was doing it under duress. I can't believe that men enjoy doing it, and I'd need a lot of convincing to persuade me otherwise."

SAM, 27

something and it's working, keep going. Sure, your tongue might get tired, but do you think blow jobs are easy?

Commandment Ten: Listen and learn

Remember, just because something sent your ex into paroxysms of lust, it doesn't mean that anyone else will enjoy it. Treat each new partner as an entirely new body (and person) to learn about. And don't go for the clichéd "drawing the alphabet with your tongue." This shows no understanding of your partner (and women can tell when you're doing it too). Instead, trail your tongue slowly over her from clit hood to perineum and left to right, and pay attention to what she likes. When her body tenses, this is generally a good sign (though it's worth checking, particularly with a new partner, that they aren't tensing in pain). Listen to her moans and groans—though don't expect them or think you're doing something wrong if she's silent. Some women are quieter than others and most women go silent just before they come. So pay attention to what she says with her body as well as her mouth.

Techniques

Now that you know what you're dealing with, you'll need some techniques so that she'll be raving about you for years to come.

Licking

Fairly basic; as the name suggests, you simply lick your partner. Try a variety of fast and slow strokes, soft and hard (always erring on the softer side though) to see which your partner likes best. Use the tip, sides, and the flat of your tongue as well as the underside.

Dribbling

Some women love feeling saliva dripping over them, and it's also handy for making sure that she's well lubricated so it delivers a double whammy.

TRY THIS NOW!

Bathe your partner then carry her through to the bedroom. Spread her legs and work your way through all the techniques. Take your time— at least five minutes per technique—and listen to her body's feedback (and her groans). Which technique is the most effective? You may find that she loves one technique when you start going down on her and another as she gets more aroused. Make a mental note of this and use your new-found knowledge in future cunnilingus sessions.

Open-mouthed sucking

Covering the whole of her clit and labia with your mouth and then softly sucking can be thrilling. If she starts going wild, don't be tempted to increase the suction. Chances are, she's writhing around because she loves exactly what you're doing so why change it?

Pulling back the clitoral hood

The clit is protected by the clit hood (much as the foreskin protects the head of the penis in uncircumcized men) However, gently pulling the hood upward then stroking the tip of the clit with your tongue can lead to particularly intense orgasms, assuming she doesn't have a hypersensitive clit. Try pressing the heel of your hand into the top of her pubes as this will naturally retract the hood for you.

Flicking

Rapid movements of the tongue over the clit or labia can help "wake it up." However, be careful not to go too wild as hard flicking can be painful.

Ovary pressing

Strange as it sounds, the ovaries can be an erogenous zone. Press into them while you're giving head—they're roughly equidistant between her navel and the side of her waist—and it can boost her orgasm.

Lubrication, lubrication, lubrication

Lube isn't just for dried up bits. It adds sensation to almost any sex act including cunnilingus. There are various types of lube that you can get: water-based, oil-based, and silicone.

It's best to avoid oil-based lubes as they make condoms rot and can be bad for genital health. Vaseline is another definite no-no. It disagrees with vaginal membranes and can lead to irritation. As to "homemade" lubes such as butter, don't even think about it. *Last Tango in Paris* has a lot to answer for too.

Water-based lubes are good all-rounders and tend to come in the greatest array of flavors: everything from strawberry to pina colada, mint to lager, and even ones that warm up on application. Some taste great while others are truly revolting: it's only by taste-testing them that you'll know which one is for you. However, you can now get sampler packs of different flavored lubricants so it needn't be expensive. Do be careful with flavored lubes though: if they contain sugar, they can encourage yeast infections, which is the last thing that you want. Water-based lubricants don't stay wet for as long as silicone-based lubes and have a tendency to get rather sticky. They can be reactivated with a water spray though, so if you keep one by the side of the bed, you'll get much more use out of said lube.

Silicone is the king of lubes. It's über-slippery and lasts for ages. However, it can't be used with silicone toys so use water-based lube if you're incorporating toy play into cunnilingus and your favorite vibrator is made out of silicone. It doesn't always taste as good as water-based lubes either: as before, taste test it to find one that you like.

Lubes come in various types of packaging: bottles, tubs, and even sprays. The best general lube packaging is a plastic squeezable flip-top lidded bottle as this means you can apply lots all in one go with ease. However, for cunnilingus, spray-on lube can be good as it applies a smaller amount and is more controllable. Tubs are best avoided for hygiene reasons.

Regardless of the lubricant that you choose, these lube tricks will show that you're the ultimate experimental oral expert.

Lick and flick
Pour some flavored lube over your partner's clit and very gently flick it with the pad of your finger while your tongue licks her labia.

In and out
Cover your fingers in lube and slide them inside her while your tongue laps her clit. A warm, moist finger is all too easy to mistake for a tongue in the heat of passion so it's also a good way to buy yourself a break if your tongue goes numb.

The drizzle
Drizzle lube over her breasts, stomach, and clit, then gradually massage her from top to bottom. Lube makes a great condom-

safe alternative to massage oil. Once she's wriggling in bliss, follow the trail of lube with your tongue and tease her all over before you eventually suck her slippery clit into your mouth.

Hot and cold

If you're into sub/dom play, alternate a warm tongue on her clit with pouring ice-cold lube straight from the fridge over her bits and rubbing it in.

Spot the tongue

Blindfold your lover and cover two fingers of each hand with lubricant. Use these to very lightly trace over either side of her labia while your tongue focuses on her clit. Swap over so your tongue is flickering over her labia and your fingers are playing with her clit. With enough practice, it should feel like she has three tongues working on her at once.

TRY THIS NOW!

Sexpert Lou Paget recommends that men tone up their tongue muscles by eating a mini fromage frais or yogurt using only their tongue. Reaching into the nooks and crannies of the pot is handy training for reaching your tongue around down below.

Go on, go on, go on

It's commonly known that women tend to take longer than men to come. As a result, you may find yourself with chronic jaw-ache mid-way through a cunnilingus session. You have various options at this point:

❀ Battle valiantly on, remembering the time she gave you a blow-job when you were hammered and kept going until the bitter end.

❀ Change position so that a different part of your jaw takes the strain.

❀ Add a vibrator to the equation.

❀ Swap to using your fingers.

If you can tell she's seconds away from coming, option one is by far the kindest. If she's stopped from coming seconds before it happens, it can scare the orgasm away altogether. However, if you sense you're going to be in it for the long haul, then any of the latter three are good options. Or hell, you could even ask her to take over for a bit. Let's face it, watching her play with herself will probably get your enthusiasm firing on all cylinders . . .

"Women don't realize how tempting it is to speed up when you're going down on them. It's like the finishing line is in sight so you put on a final spurt of speed!"

PETER, 29

Troubleshooting

There are of course problems you may encounter when going down, but most of these are easily dealt with when you're prepared for what can go wrong.

When she doesn't come

Although oral sex is one of the easiest ways to make a woman come, it's by no means guaranteed. Stress, tiredness, excessive alcohol, or even something as simple as having distracting music on in the background can all make it hard for a woman to reach climax. However, it could be that the reason she's not coming is that you're either going at it so hard she fears for her clit, or that you're changing your style so often that she can't get into the rhythm. You may be positioning your hands in such a way that they dig in uncomfortably or it could be that your stubble is chafing her. If things seem to be taking a long time, start off by pulling back and going gently. Ask

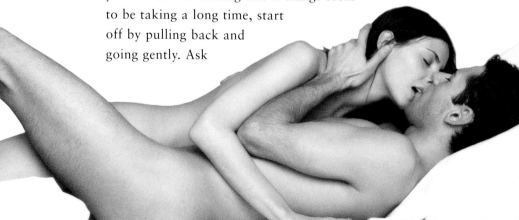

her if you're doing anything wrong so that she has "permission" to correct your technique. If that still doesn't work, don't see it as a failure: just ask if you can take a break for a bit and cuddle up to your partner. You can always use some nifty fingerwork to keep her horny. Alternatively, using a bullet-style toy on her clit while you lick her will probably help speed things along.

When you get a hair in your throat

Don't try to struggle on valiantly: you'll only end up choking. When you feel a hair in your mouth, discreetly spit it out onto your hand—or for a sneaky trick, spit on her clit. This will add extra lube—never a bad thing, as you know—and get rid of the offending hair in one move. Do check your partner doesn't object to this type of behavior though: some women may feel degraded by it. Then again, sometimes that can be hot . . .

If getting hairs in your throat is a common occurrence then consider asking your lover very nicely if she'd be up for shaving her pubes—or at least trimming them. If you promise you'll lavish her with lots more oral attention, she'll probably consider it worth the effort.

When she squeezes too hard

It's all too easy for a woman to get caught up in the heat of the moment and clench her thighs together so tightly that you fear you'll get a broken neck. While you can ask your partner not to do it, controlling orgasmic bliss is kind of tricky. Instead, opt for tying your lover up spread-eagled, if you both like a bit of bondage, or putting your elbows in between her thighs while you go down on her so that she'll be straining against them rather than your face. Alternatively, enjoy the submissive thrill of being stifled—some men really get off on it.

When you don't like the taste

A clean and healthy vagina should taste great. However, the taste of vaginal juices can change across a women's menstrual cycle and sometimes it's less tasty than usual. If this is the case, use saliva to "dilute" the taste. With copious dribbling you should be able to mask any unpleasantness. Alternatively, experiment with flavored lubricants or chocolate sauce. Just make sure that your lover washes thoroughly afterward to avoid yeast infections.

Dos and Don'ts

For her

1. Do show you love it. 66 percent of men rate their partner's reaction as the top turn-on when they perform oral.
2. Don't clamp your legs together so tightly it limits your partner's movement.
3. Do wash beforehand. Clean bits are nicer to be near.
4. Don't forget to comb through your pubes when you get out of the bath to get rid of any potentially choking stragglers.
5. Do say if something isn't working—how else will he know what to do?

For him

1. Don't go down for 30 seconds and expect her to be grateful.
2. Do ask what she likes. If she finds it hard to explain, have a "training session" where you try different things.
3. Don't treat cunnilingus as a trading card—"I'll do it for you if you go down on me."
4. Do remember that oral sex during periods is a higher risk activity STD-wise so make sure you use a dental dam.
5. Don't go down after you've had sex using a condom with spermicide. It will make your tongue go numb.

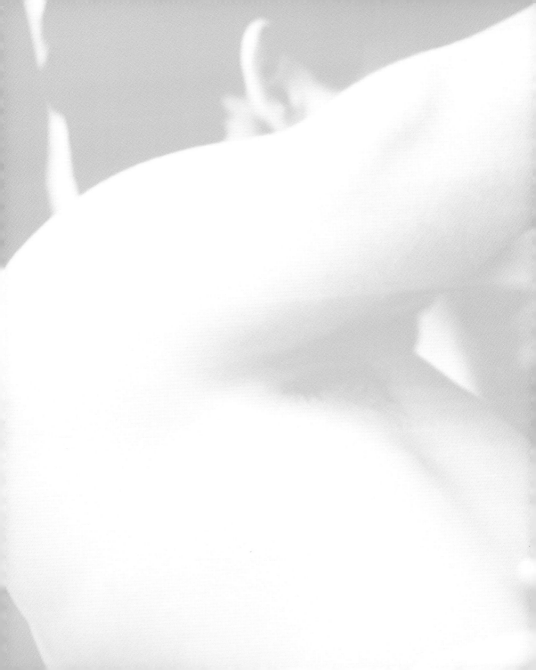

PLEASURING
A MAN

When it comes to pleasuring a man, you've already got one major

advantage: oral is one of most men's favorite sex acts, and merely

initiating it will already mark you out as one hot woman.

3

A load of cock: The anatomy of the penis

To properly pleasure a penis, you need to know how it works. Although it might seem simple—touch it, lick it, feel it grow hard—there's more to a man's member than you may think. Not all parts of the penis are created equal: some respond instantly to pleasure while other bits still like being caressed but won't work as many wonders. Knowing where the über-erogenous zones are—even the ones that are hidden—is the first step to being a phenomenal fellatrix. So it's worth getting to grips (ahem) with the basic anatomy.

Ask your man to spread his legs then sit between them so that you've got the best view. Get him hard so that you can see the penis in its best possible state.

Starting at the top, you've got the glans: the rounded bit also known as the head of the penis. This is one of the most sensitive bits of the penis: the equivalent of a woman's clitoris. Focusing your attention here will reap the most rewards.

In the tip of the glans is the urethra, which he urinates through and ejaculates from. Some men find stimulation of the urethral opening (aka meatus) intense while others find it a massive turn off. Try running your tongue lightly around the urethra to gauge his response: if he likes it, you can try darting your tongue lightly into the urethra. However, don't stick anything down there as it can get stuck and cause intense pain.

At the bottom of the glans is the coronal ridge. This is also incredibly sensitive: try running your tongue around it when your man's aroused to see how intense the pleasure can be.

Continuing down, next comes the frenulum. This is the stringy bit on the base of the glans, and is one of the ultimate male erogenous zones. Try lightly flicking it with your tongue, softly sucking on it, or letting your thumb rub over it while your tongue works on his glans. If a man is uncircumcized, this is the point at which his foreskin attaches so you can also try running your tongue underneath his foreskin. Go gently though: while this can be phenomenal for some men, others find it too much. It's also possible to break the frenulum, if you're rough, which can result in blood loss and extreme pain so save your maximum suction for stimulating the shaft—which is the bit that you'll get to next.

The shaft forms the bulk of the penis (unless the man is particularly unlucky size-wise). It's less sensitive than the head, but responds well to firm strokes and suction. However, some men do have extremely sensitive areas on their shaft so it's worth exploring your man thoroughly with lubed-up fingers to see whether he has any particularly erogenous zones that you can use to your advantage.

"My wife loves giving me oral, but hates to taste my come, so when she goes down on me she purses her lips real tight when I'm about to come. She looks sexy as hell when she does it, I get to shoot my load where I want to, and she doesn't have to swallow. As long as there's a box of tissues and a glass of orange juice nearby, she's happy."

DAN, 38

Many women think that that's it, overlooking anything below that level but this is a massive mistake: the scrotum and balls can both be erogenous zones, once you've reassured your man that you're not going to squeeze too hard or play too roughly. Try sucking the balls into your mouth (known as teabagging if you approach from underneath him). Some men like it if you suck them one at a time, others like the sensation of having both balls in your mouth. Alternatively, if he's too nervous about having his family jewels so near to your teeth, or has balls that are too big to fit into your mouth, try lapping at the skin of the scrotum between his balls or softly sucking it into your mouth.

Finally, there's the perineum. This is the area between his balls and his anus, also known as the "t'aint" because it "ain't his butt and it ain't his penis." Running your tongue over this area firmly, or pressing into it with the heel of your hand or (short-nailed) fingertips can indirectly stimulate his prostate gland (of which more later) from the outside, making it ideal if your man is nervous about anal play.

Although most men would be more than happy if you merely paid attention to all the above areas, a bit of sensual exploration can enhance the experience even more. The only way to find these erogenous zones is to explore, so make sure that you set aside time to get to know every inch of your man rather than assuming that they're all the same. Once you know where to touch, it's time to move on to what to do: welcome to the blow job basics.

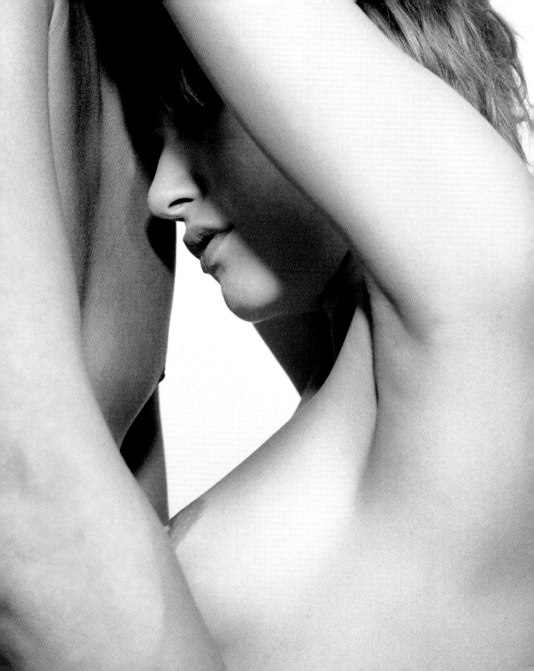

The blow job basics

Once you know what's going on down there, there are a few golden rules to remember before you go down.

Basic One: Cover those teeth

There's a time and a place for nibbling, and when you've got your man's penis between your lips, it's most definitely not the time. Make sure that you have your teeth covered with your lips before you get carried away, and if your man starts thrusting away too vigorously, don't be afraid to pull back—all too many penile injuries have been caused by overenthusiastic action. The only time to get your teeth involved is if a man asks you to, and even then, go gently.

Basic Two: Use your hands

Just because it's called oral sex, it doesn't mean that it's exclusively oral. Using your hands will enhance the sensation for him, speed his climax along, and give your mouth a break if you start to get jaw ache. Try masturbating his shaft while your tongue circles his glans, rubbing your thumb over his frenulum while his penis is inside your mouth, or playing with his balls while you deep throat him.

Basic Three: The wetter the better

Lube isn't just for women. Using lots of saliva or, better, adding a dash of flavored lube will help everything glide more easily. This is particularly important if your man is circumcized as he won't produce as much natural lubrication. Take your pick from strawberry, chocolate, or pina colada, to name just a few.

Basic Four: Ask for it

Or better yet, beg. Most men are of the opinion that women don't enjoy administering oral sex. As such, if you make the first move, they're likely to think:

- Way-hey, it's my lucky night.
- She is such a hot woman.
- Where did that erection come from? It wasn't there 20 seconds ago.

And thus the warming up is done for you. A woman who initiates oral sex will never be short of a man.

Basic Five: Show your enthusiasm

Of course, Basic Four only works if you then show that you're loving it once you get down to business. There's no point sucking a man half-heartedly: he'll feel like it's a chore for you and you'll be down there for hours while he wrestles with the

"I love coming in my girlfriend's hair, but it's obviously not a spur-of-the-moment thing to do, so on Saturday mornings I go down on her while she sleeps, until she wakes up, incredibly horny, and tosses me off in her hair. Then we both take a shower and I wash it all out."

OLI, 29

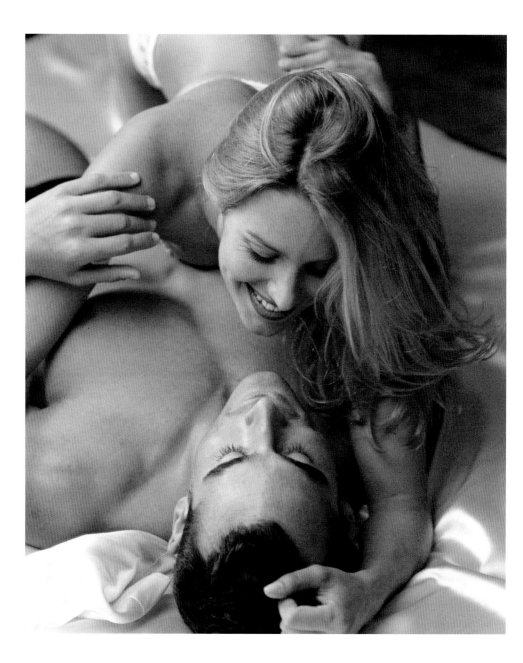

dilemma of "I feel guilty she's doing something she doesn't like, but it feels so good . . ."

Basic Six: Be an explorer

Don't just stick to sucking the penis. Let your hands and tongue roam over your man's balls, perineum, chest, and inner thighs. Don't go for prostate massage without warning though. While it works for some men, others (quite rightly) take offense at having a finger stuck there as a "surprise."

Basic Seven: Keep on going

Yes, giving a blow job can sometimes seem like it's taking forever but women don't exactly come in seconds, so be patient. If your partner is under the influence of drink, spend more time on masturbating him before you move on to oral sex. Although a blow job doesn't have to be taken to completion every time, it's good manners to keep on going until the (often) bitter end.

Basic Eight: The look of lust

Men are visual creatures so give him something to look at and he'll enjoy himself a lot more. If you're relatively shy, try just looking him in the eye as you suck him. If you're a little more confident, play with your breasts and if you're wild and willing to try anything, get a toy involved and play with yourself as you suck him, making sure that you're in a position that allows him the best view. A mirror can be a handy oral accomplice . . .

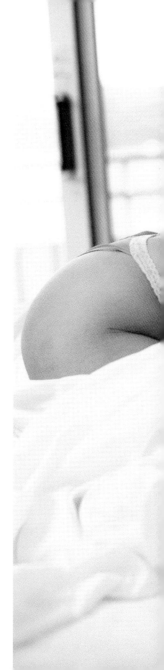

Basic Nine: Talk with your mouth full

You may have been told that it's bad manners but the occasional comment during oral sex can be helpful: think "God, I love sucking you," rather than, "I've been thinking, the bathroom needs grouting." If he's taking a long time to come, throwing in a quick "I want to taste your come" will probably prove "I want" does get in certain situations.

Basic Ten: Take it like a woman

Yes, it's the old spit or swallow debate. If you really hate the taste of semen then don't feel obliged to swallow. Either discreetly spit it into a tissue you've left by the side of the bed, along with a glass of juice to drink, or better yet, ask him to ejaculate over your breasts or face instead. This is a move often used in porn films and, as such, is likely to make him think that you're one hot woman. Just remember to close your eyes if you go for the latter option.

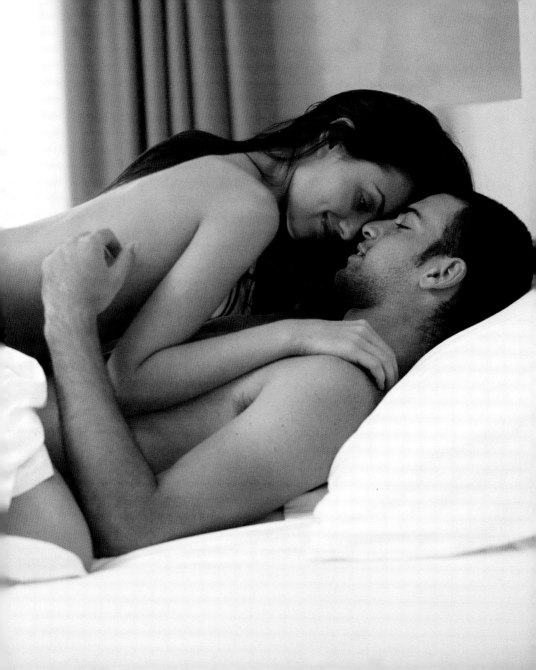

TIPS FOR HER FROM HIM
Spit or swallow: the great debate

OK, this is one of the most meaningless debates in the entire realm of sexuality, but let's drag it out into the open once and for all. Is coming into a woman's mouth or on her face an incredible turn-on for men? Yes. You only have to look at the millions of porn scenes floating around the Internet to know that's true.

In the real world, however, things are a little more complicated. A girl who swallows is either seen as incredibly sensuous, or a bit of a slut. Usually both. There's still a huge stigma over ejaculating in someone's mouth, and it's not likely to go away any time soon. Personally, I can't see what the fuss is about. I don't care where I come, as long as I do. You could have it in your mouth, in your hair, on your tits, in your hand, up your elbow, over a dartboard, in a matchbox—anywhere you like, as long as it's out.

If your partner likes the taste of sperm (and a lot of women do, particularly if you maintain a good diet and keep yourself clean), then good. If she's willing to take it into her mouth before letting it out, good. If she lets you shoot your load down her face, neck, breasts, or anywhere else, good. Are you detecting a pattern here? It's all good. I've been with women who swallowed, women who spat, and women who did neither, and I can't recall getting extra pleasure from one group over the other; what I can remember is what they did to get me there in the first place.

Personally, there is nothing sexier than being jerked off into an open mouth inches away from the tip of my penis (with complimentary pleading eyes and encouraging noises). But when that triggers the impending ejaculation, it's all about her from then on in, and she has the total right to direct my dick anywhere she likes. Doesn't matter to me— I'm already coming.

And, to be totally honest with you, I'd much rather do that than have to see my partner spit it out into a hanky, or have her ruining the post-coital afterglow by dashing to the bathroom to gargle with mouthwash for half an hour, or—even worse—slapping a ban on oral because I made her retch or choke. The key to perfect oral sex, you see, is trust— as a man, I'm trusting one of the most delicate parts of my body to my partner's mouth (which has teeth, after all, and the capability to harm it by biting it or blowing down it). Therefore, she has to trust me not to hurt or offend her by shoving it down her throat, poking her in the face, or ejaculating anywhere that's off-limits. And if trust breaks down on either side, the oral sex will be nothing more than an unsatisfactory token gesture.

Techniques

Once you know where to touch, it's time to move on to technique. After you've mastered a few basics, up the pace with some advanced techniques and he'll be gibbering in lust. Simply adding lube, changing your suction, or flickering your tongue over his most sensitive parts can make all the difference.

Licking

By far the simplest and least tongue-intensive motion, licking can be used to tease a man into hardness, keep him on the edge deliciously, or add extra sophistication while deep-throating—just keep your tongue licking as you let him slide to the back of your throat. Seeing you enthusiastically lapping his nether regions is sure to drive a man wild. As recommended in cunnilingus, use the tip, sides, and the flat of your tongue as well as the underside as they all offer different sensations.

Dribbling

Dribbling is a classic porn star trick used to add extra lubrication and make things move more easily. For the full X-rated effect, do it from a distance, and alternate it with hard spitting. Dirty talk is a good addition to this.

Open-mouthed sucking

Sometimes it's best to tease a man, particularly if you've got him tied up. This is where open-mouthed sucking comes into its own. Put your mouth around his penis then simply breathe, letting him feel the warmth of your breath. Keep your mouth as wide open as possible so that he doesn't brush the sides. Then, when he's all but given up on the idea that you're ever going to suck him, put your lips around him and slide as far down his member as you can in one move. Don't be surprised if he comes immediately though.

Hoovering

Suction is intensive on your jaw muscles but feels so good for most men that it's harsh to omit it from your repertoire. Simply put his penis between your lips then suck, alternating between soft and hard "hoovering." If you get tired, swap to using your hand while you lick him instead.

Flicking

Using your tongue to flick the most sensitive parts of the penis can be wonderfully pleasurable. Focus your attentions on the frenulum, the vein along the underside of the penis, and the tip of the glans.

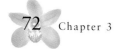

Lubrication, lubrication, lubrication

Lubrication is an essential addition to any sex act—and not just for women. A well-lubricated hand sliding up a man's shaft while soft lips tease the head will give him one of life's ultimate pleasures. Be creative about the way that you apply it too—it can enhance the experience even more.

Obviously, if you're choosing a lubricant to use during oral sex it makes sense to choose a flavored one. If you can't find any in your local sex shop, check out one of the numerous online sex shops. If that's not an option, choose the most basic lube you can: spermicide and Nonoxynol-9 taste horrid and numb the tongue, so you don't want to go for a lube that contains either of them for oral sex.

TRY THIS NOW!

The perfect way to boost a man's confidence is with a long, lingering oral session. Start by lightly kissing from the tip of his glans right down his shaft to his perineum. Then work your way back up his shaft, this time letting your tongue lap up the vein of his penis as you go. Flicker it from side to side, then capture the glans between your lips and swirl your tongue around the coronal ridge in a circular motion. Then slip his glans between your lips once more and flutter your tongue over the frenulum. When you feel his penis start to pulse move your lips down to the base of his penis, taking the head as far down your throat as is comfortable.

Breast friend

Cover your breasts in lubricant then slide his penis between them to get it thoroughly slathered in lube. Lean forward to lick the tip of his penis as he slides forward. (NB. you may not even get to full oral sex if you choose this option: there's a good chance he'll come before you get your mouth full.)

High hopes

Hold the lube high above your man's penis and pour it from above, using the other hand to masturbate his shaft. This is a messy way to apply lube, but that can be half the fun.

Rear action

Lube up your buttocks and get your man to slide in between them, with his penis aiming upward toward your back rather than downward into your nether regions. Do make sure that you tell him that you're not attempting to initiate anal sex though: a man can get the wrong idea, after all . . .

The masseuse

Give your lover a massage using lubricant rather than oil. Just make sure that you add extra when you get to his groin, so that there's maximum slipperiness. Follow the trail of the lube with your tongue afterward and he'll be blissed out.

Troubleshooting

Of course, oral sex isn't always fun to administer: gagging, "funky" spunk, and thoughtless lovers who fail to understand that a hand on the back of the head really isn't helping can all lead to a less than perfect night. As such, you need to know how to troubleshoot these issues and more.

When he doesn't come

Even though most men would list blow jobs as one of their favorite sex acts, there's no guarantee that it will lead to orgasm every time. Many men complain that they can't reach climax during oral sex, particularly if they masturbate regularly and are used to the somewhat firmer grip of their own hand. Remember that patience is a virtue and there's a reasonable chance that your man's spent hours trying to get you to come, so it's only fair to return the favor. If, however, you're beginning to fear lockjaw, you have various options:

- Change position. If you're kneeling between his legs, try moving round to approach from the side instead. This will mean you can rest your head on his stomach to give your neck a break. Men tend to enjoy the view of a woman's bits, as their fondness for porn demonstrates, so giving him a graphic view may well help.

- Use your hand rather than your mouth, throwing in the occasional lick so that he doesn't think you've gone off the way that he tastes. Even if you have.

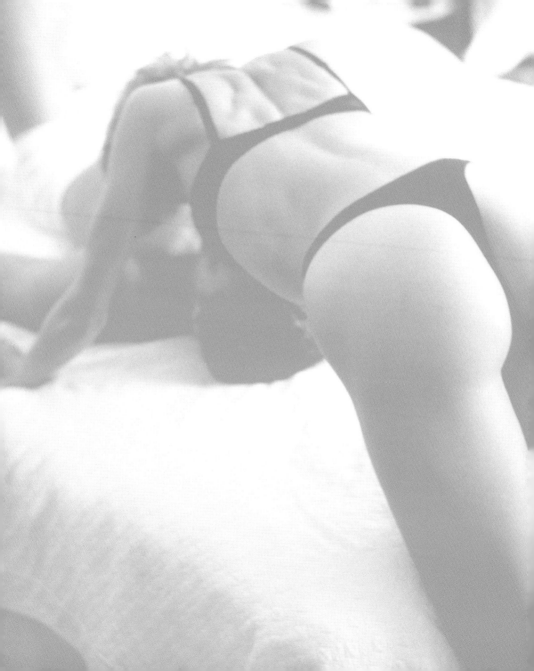

❀ Ask him to masturbate over your face. Thus, he does the work and you get the "reward." Or, to be more accurate, you both do.

❀ Ask him to masturbate while you put on a masturbation show for him. This delivers an orgasm for you and a visual delight for him at the same time.

❀ Suggest that you move on to having penetrative sex. If he's having a hard time coming, hard doggie-style is probably your best bet to do the job.

❀ If you really can't go on any longer, apologize and say that you're going to have to take a break. Just remember to be more understanding the next time that he has to stop when he's going down on you.

When you start to gag

Generally speaking, if you're gagging it's because he's pushing too hard. The logical solution is to remove his hands from the back of your head or press down on his hips to quell the overenthusiastic thrusting. You can also train your gag reflex, of which more later when we get to deep-throat techniques. However, you shouldn't be expected to be a sword swallower every time, so pull away if gets uncomfortable. Yes, throat-gagging blow jobs may feature in most porn films nowadays but the women administering them are getting paid for it. You're no less of a woman if you can't take a full eight inches—or even a full five inches—into your throat, so have the confidence to push him away.

When he puts his hand on the back of your head

See above. Explain to your man that hand on back of head equals gagging which can equal vomiting. Unless he's exceptionally kinky, that should be enough to do the trick. It's probably best to point out that you dislike hands on your head before you're getting down to it though—otherwise all that talk of vomit could spoil the mood.

When his come tastes "funky"

If a man's semen tastes unpleasant—or "funky," as Samantha in *Sex and the City* so eloquently described it—you need to take the long term approach. Smoking, drinking, eating curry or asparagus, and having a generally unhealthy diet can all affect the taste of semen. Encourage your man to eat lots of fruit: pineapple juice and strawberries are both highly recommended. If he hasn't ejaculated for a while it can also increase the bitterness of his semen (and possibly his attitude) so encourage him to masturbate regularly (and have lots of sex too). Short-term, all you can do is take it as far down your throat as possible so that it passes over the minimum taste buds, or grab a glass of juice at the first available opportunity.

When you get a pubic hair stuck in your throat

See "troubleshooting" section in Chapter Two. And yes, there's nothing wrong with asking a man to shave down below, particularly if he expects you to trim your bush.

Dos and Don'ts

For her

1. Don't just suck. Use a variety of techniques and let your hands rove around his erogenous zones for the ultimate blow job.

2. Do be enthusiastic. OK, so a lackluster blow job is still better than no blow job at all but if you show that you love it, not only will you have more fun—it's amazing how quickly acting enthusiastically can turn into genuine enthusiasm when you see how much your partner's enjoying himself—but it's also likely to take a lot less time.

3. Don't try to fit it all down your throat if you're not comfortable with deep throat techniques. Yes, it can enhance things for the guy but not to the extent that it's worth choking yourself for.

4. Do keep flavored lubricant, a hair band (if you have long hair), tissues, and a glass of juice near to the bed. That way you've got all you need to administer great oral sex, hold your hair back to present the best view, deal with any pubic hairs that get trapped in your throat, and rinse out your mouth afterward if you're not a fan of the taste of semen.

5. Don't use your teeth. Yes, it's been said before but it really is an important rule to remember.

For him

1. Don't put your hands on the back of her head. It will encourage the gagging reflex and unless you're living out a role play with your partner as submissive, it's unlikely she'll enjoy it. Even if you are indulging in power games, be careful that you don't choke her too much. Smeared mascara may look hot in a kinky kind of way but choking fits just aren't fun.

2. Do warn your lover before you come. That way she can prepare to swallow. More to the point, it's only polite.

3. Don't use the line "While you're down there," every time a woman is on her knees. We've heard it before. So many times.

4. Do be careful about where you grip your partner when she's administering oral. Although finger-shaped bruises can be hot the next day, if you grip your lover so tightly around the shoulders that she's in pain, it's unlikely she'll be enthusiastic about doing it again.

5. Don't promise you won't come in her mouth then go back on your word. Yes, it's tricky holding back your orgasm and can be tempting to "go with the flow" but if you break a promise, you're likely to suffer—not least from lack of fellatio in future.

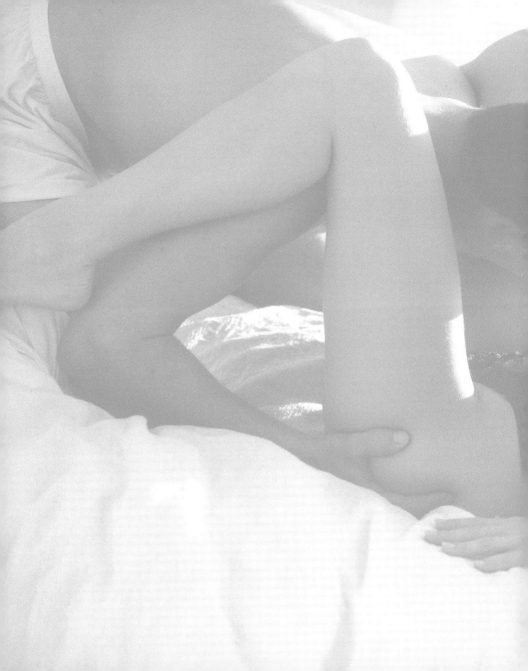

ORAL SEX POSITIONS

As with all things sexual, variety is the spice of life so it's important to mix things up as often as you can by experimenting with different oral sex positions. All of them give you access to different erogenous zones meaning that no two oral sex experiences need ever be the same, though they'll all be equally as good.

4

Ladies first: Cunnilingus positions

You might feel smug now that you've got to grips with what to do, honed your techniques, and experimented with lube. However, don't think that you can just relax, content that your oral mastery will blow your lover away. You need to vary your routine so that she doesn't always know exactly what's coming, and that means trying some new positions. An advantage of multiple positions is that you can change from one to another when you start to get tired: it's amazing the difference that moving around can make to your energy levels.

Read on for the top cunnilingus positions to try. Don't expect every position to hit the spot with every partner, but by having a selection to choose from, you can guarantee that you'll be able to find something that will do the trick for you and her.

TRY THIS NOW!

Pick three cunnilingus positions that you've never tried before, and ask your man to try all three in one session. Make a note of which ones you most enjoy and why. Once you've finished, tell him so that next time he knows what to do.

Worship her

This position puts the woman in charge—it allows plenty of scope for you to grab your partner's head and pull it deeper into you, if that's something that both of you enjoy doing.

The woman sits on a chair with the man kneeling between her legs. Depending on the sort of chair that you choose, the woman can either spread her legs then hook her ankles around the front two legs of the chair, or throw her legs over the arms of an armchair. The man then leans forward and starts licking.

Pros

Both versions of this position allow easy access to the vagina, and the latter makes it easy for the man to administer analingus too. It also leaves both of the man's hands free to stimulate the woman's vagina and breasts. You can easily incorporate a toy in this position. Some women may also get a dominant thrill from being pleasured in this way.

Cons

Some men feel uncomfortable about assuming a submissive role. It can also hurt the man's knees if he's down there for a long time, so remember to put a cushion down first. Some women feel too exposed in this position and would prefer to try something a little less exhibitionistic.

Bobbing for apples

This is one of the classic positions and is ideal for a lazy
Sunday morning (for the woman at least—the man has to work
fairly hard).

The woman lies on her back and the man kneels or lies
between her thighs with his head, fairly obviously, at groin
level. He then starts licking.

Pros

This is very relaxing for the woman and gives the man easy
access to her clitoris, breasts, and vagina. It's also easy to get
fingers involved in this position.

Cons

This can be quite tiring for the man. It can also lead to
arguments about duvet positioning, particularly in winter when
the woman wants to stay warm while she's being pleasured but
the man risks suffocation if he's covered by the duvet. If you're
into anal play, you won't be able to reach it as easily as in
other positions.

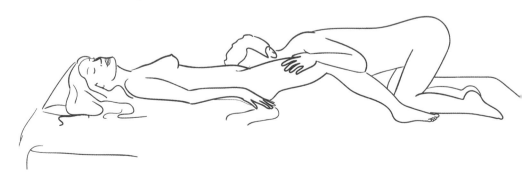

Sit on my face and wiggle

It may have a comedy name but this position is far from a joke. Many women find this one of the most effective positions for reaching climax, and a fair few men love the submissive thrill that they get from being smothered by their partner's most intimate parts.

As the name suggests, the man lies down and the woman then straddles his face. She can then grind over his lips, tongue, and even nose until she reaches climax.

Pros

This is a great position for women who have a hard time coming. It allows the woman full control and offers clitoral stimulation through the nose and chin as well as the more usual tongue and lips. Some women may also get a dominant thrill from being pleasured in this way.

Cons

Some women may find it harder to climax with their legs tensed. It can also be all too easy to inadvertently squash a man if you get carried away, and hampering someone's breathing just isn't cool.

Hoodwinked

If a woman has a particularly sensitive clitoris, she may find direct clitoral stimulation too intense. If so, this position which focuses attention on the clitoral hood is just what you need.

The woman lies on her back. The man then kneels to one side of her and approaches her clitoris from a new angle. Rather than aiming for the clitoral tip, he should work only on the clitoral hood unless asked otherwise.

Pros

It helps you avoid hurting a sensitive partner. It can also offer a fantastic sense of anticipation, as you avoid the sensitive clitoral tip until your partner is totally aroused. It's a good position to use if you plan on involving sex toys as well.

Cons

This position can give the man neck ache if it's sustained for extended amounts of time. Some women find that it doesn't offer enough stimulation, and others may find it impersonal as there's less body contact than in other positions.

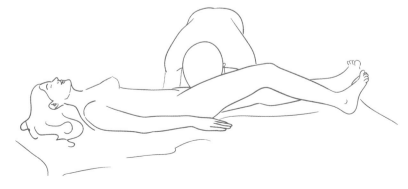

Reary good

And of course, there's always rear entry if you're looking for something a little different.

The woman gets on all fours, doggie-style. The man then kneels behind her to lap at her folds.

Pros

This position allows easy clitoral stimulation, anal stimulation, and vaginal penetration. Some men find the view particularly arousing.

Cons

Some women may feel vulnerable in such an explicit position—and this position isn't advised if the woman's just eaten chilli.

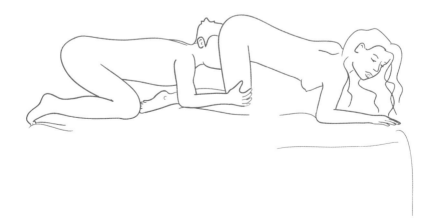

Over and above

If you're looking for a position with mutual benefit, this one is a potential winner.

The woman lies on her back and the man then kneels above her, facing her feet, with his lips at groin level.

Pros

All you need to do to turn this into soixante-neuf is get the woman to lift her head. The man can brush his penis between the woman's breasts as he's pleasuring her too, making it a good compromise position if the woman wants oral sex and the man's not in the mood. It gives easy access to the clitoral tip, and it's also easy to spread the woman's labia in this position. Some women may also get a submissive thrill from being pleasured in this way.

Cons

It's tricky for the man to insert his fingers or a toy in the woman from this position, and the view isn't particularly appealing for the women, unless she's a fan of hanging testicles and a hairy anus.

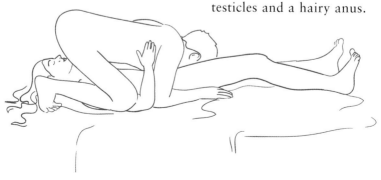

Bed head

You don't always have to lie in the bed to get great orgasms. Sometimes the edge of the bed can be the perfect location.

The woman lies on the bottom of the bed with her feet on the floor and genitals at the edge. The man kneels on the floor to administer oral.

Pros

This position offers women a dominant thrill and gives the man easy access to her genitals, vagina and anus (depending on how far over the edge of the bed she positions herself). She also gets to stay warm under the duvet while enjoying oral.

Cons

This isn't the most comfortable position for the man but he may get a submissive kick from it. Putting a pillow underneath his knees may help.

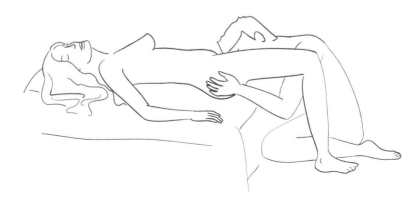

TIPS FOR HER FROM HIM
The downsides of giving head

It goes without saying that everything about cunnilingus is great, but for men, there are a lot of drawbacks; none more so than when you're a novice. The first few experiences can literally make or break your development in that particular field of foreplay.

Complicated techniques

The thing about cunnilingus is that it's—for want of a better expression—incredibly difficult to get your head around at first. By comparison, fellatio is a breeze; here's my penis, get your mouth around it, bob up and down for a bit. Simple. Female genitals, on the other hand, look (and are) remarkably complicated by comparison, as well as being a tad scary for the newcomer.

Lack of education

The situation's made even worse when you consider that the three main fonts of carnal knowledge—Dads, sex education lessons, and porn movies—teach you absolutely nothing on the subject. Alright, maybe porn teaches you something, but seeing as that "something" goes along the lines of "flick your tongue in the general direction of her groin for a few seconds before she sucks your dick for 20 minutes," there's nothing of educational value to be gleaned. Which means the first time you go down—more often than not with someone who is just as experienced as you, i.e., not very—it's probably going to be a less than gratifying moment.

Communicate

It's only when you meet a partner who knows what she likes (and isn't shy to communicate it) that you really hit your stride. So if you're female and dealing with a relative novice, don't hold back on the chatter—tell him what to do, how it feels, and when he should stop and move on.

Time and dedication

Another huge problem that men have with cunnilingus is the fact that it takes a long time to get right, and even then you're not guaranteed the pay-off of a female orgasm. Men, being the goal-orientated animals they are, can equate their partners not being able to climax through their oral attempts as a failure, and not the essential part of foreplay it can be. There's an easy (yet sneaky) solution; simply demand to be taken, right now. His ego will live to fight another day, and he'll feel he's discovered a new tool in his armory, and will want to use it again and again.

Fears and insecurities

As for his fears about smell and taste, well, women can't (and shouldn't) attempt to alter it—it's supposed to taste and smell like a vagina, and in a very short while he'll discover that it's an easily acquirable taste. As long as both of you maintain a decent standard of hygiene, there's nothing to worry about. Oh, and if you want him to go at it for a sufficient length of time, you ought to consider a comfy position to get into, as lying face-down on a bed for a considerable length of time is a real strain on those neck muscles. A pillow propped under the bum is good. Two are better.

Head boy: Fellatio positions

Of course, different positions aren't just beneficial for cunnilingus, men like a little variety as well. By changing the angle from which you approach fellatio, you can increase access to a man's perineum or prostate, allow him access to your breasts or bits, or simply give him a sexy view. Different positions are also handy if you start to get tired. A change really can be as good as a rest. Just make sure that you don't change pace when your man's nearing the edge of return—unless, of course, you feel like teasing him to distraction and want to make him wait . . .

TRY THIS NOW!

Standing 69s are probably the gold medal event of oral sex—but more often than not you require a strong male, an agile female, and a lot of balance to carry it off. So if you want to try out a similar experience without doing yourself an injury (and have a strong enough armchair), try it with the male in a seated position, and the female resting her knees on the top of the armchair. Not only does it give the female full upside-down access, she can also take a breather by resting her hands on his thighs.

Begging for it

This is a classic position, much beloved of porn directors and dominant men.

The man stands and the woman kneels in front of him.

Pros

This is incredibly easy to get into, can give the man a dominant thrill or the woman a submissive kick, and allows easy access to the balls, perineum, and anus.

Cons

The woman's knees may get sore, in which case a cushion can help. The man may get carried away and thrust too deeply in this position, making the woman gag, and some women may feel demeaned in this position.

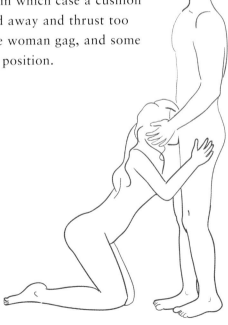

Sideways suckstress

Changing the angle of approach can lead to different sensations as new erogenous zones are stimulated.

The man lies on his back. The woman kneels to one side of him and fellates him.

Pros

If the man likes anal play, this position allows easy access for toys. It also allows easy access to the balls and perineum.

Cons

This can make the woman's neck ache, and if a guy is particularly thick, it can be tricky to fit it into the woman's mouth from this angle.

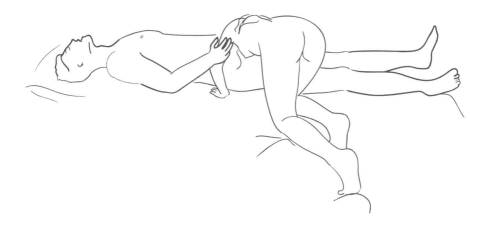

Admiring the view

Men tend to get aroused by visual stimulation so this position offers the best of both worlds—oral sex and a sexy view.

The woman straddles the man, facing toward his feet, then fellates him.

Pros

The man has a great view of the woman's vagina and anus, and can play with her at the same time if he wants to. Should you decide to move into the 69 position, all the woman needs to do is lower her bits onto the man's face.

Cons

Some women may feel too exposed in this position. Approaching the penis from above can be a tricky angle to maintain, and may lead to teeth scraping across the penis. It can also make the woman's neck ache.

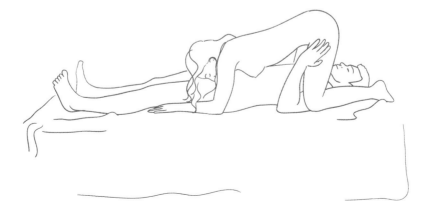

Lazy lady

If a woman's feeling tired, she may want a relaxing position to fellate in (if she's feeling up for it at all). This provides the ideal solution.

The woman lies on her back with pillows under her head to ensure that she's at the right angle for easy penetration. The man then thrusts into her mouth.

Pros

This can make the man feel dominant, and allows the woman to focus on sucking rather than bobbing her head. It's also ideal if you both like the idea of the man ejaculating on the woman's face.

Cons

It can be easy for a man to get carried away and thrust too deeply, inciting the gag reflex.

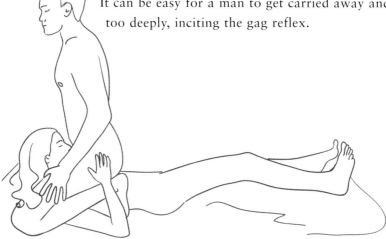

Chairman of the board

If a man has "sexy secretary" fantasies, this position is just
what you need.

   The man sits on a chair and the woman kneels at his feet,
fellating him.

Pros

This is ideal if the man is dominant and woman is submissive.
It allows easy access to the balls, and anus if the man moves to
the edge of the chair.

Cons

Again, this position isn't easy on the knees, you may
want to put a cushion down.

Sofa, so good

What could be better than a blow job during the commercial breaks when you're watching a film?

The man sits on a sofa. The woman sits next to him, bending over to take his penis in her mouth.

Pros

It's quick and easy to get into, and gives the man a sense of decadent pleasure.

Cons

This can be painful on the woman's neck. If the man takes too long to come and the commericial break ends, you may find a particularly scary or gruesome scene in a film can spoil the mood. Or worse, doesn't.

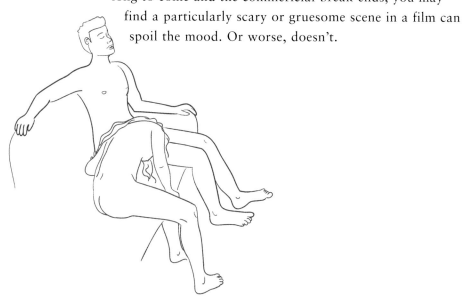

You spin me right round

A favorite in modern porn films, this isn't the easiest of positions to get in to but certainly has "wow" factor.

The man stands up near the edge of a bed. The woman then does a handstand on the bed, and hooks her legs around the man's neck, and arms around his waist. She then fellates him upside-down, while he uses his arms to support her lower back.

Pros

It's certainly impressive if you can pull this one off (as long as you don't actually pull it off!). The man can control depth of penetration by raising and lowering his partner.

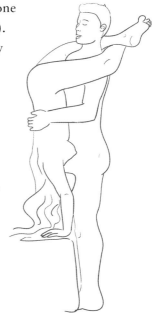

Cons

It's almost impossible to get into, and the man needs exceptionally strong legs. Holding the woman's weight may also make it difficult for the man to concentrate on the job in, er, mouth.

TIPS FOR HER FROM HIM
What men look for in a fellatio position

Men have the merest of requirements receiving head; they want to be
comfortable, to have their partner's bits within reach, to be able to see
what their partner is doing, a mix of techniques, their partner to cover all
genital bases, and a modicum of control over when and where they
ejaculate. Oh, and they want their partners to look as if they're enjoying
themselves while they're doing all those things. OK, so maybe we lied
about the "merest" bit; there are a lot of requirements to fulfil in order to
achieve the perfect blow job, so let's break them down one by one . . .

Comfort

If you want him to come, you have to give him the opportunity to
simultaneously relax and concentrate—so him in a sitting position with
you between his legs and on your knees is a good place to start (some
men prefer a standing position, but others find it uncomfortable, mainly
because they tend to hunch over at the point of climax). However, make
sure your comfort isn't compromised, especially on the knees. Another
good position involves him propped up on the bed; it's a bit less
dominant, more comfortable for both partners, and also fulfils the next
requirement very nicely . . .

Strokability

If he's flat out on the bed or floor, you have greater access to his penis
and balls. More importantly, he has greater access to you—so not only

do you feel the benefit of some much-deserved attention, he has something to do which helps him relax and really get into it.

Techniques

A man can really get used to having the same part of his penis manipulated over and over again. No, really. It's a common fact that women love blended orgasms (where more than one erogenous zone is being manipulated), and the same goes for men. Combine the caressing of his balls while you're deep-throating him, or run your tongue all the way up the underside of his shaft with a well-licked thumb over the head, and he'll be putty in your hands.

Enjoyment

If you show the slightest flicker of discomfort, distaste, or flat-out going-through-the-motions, he'll notice it and will give up. You don't have to screech like a banshee while you're doing it or act like a fake porn starlet—just take your time, and be as coquettish as you like. Men are absolute suckers for eye contact—one well-timed glance can be the equivalent of two minutes of frenzied sucking.

Control

If he's getting ready to come and he takes his cock back, don't be offended. He's not saying that you can't finish the job—he wants to draw out the experience for as long as possible, and he also knows just how much punishment his penis can take to bring him off.

Top positions for mutual oral

Then of course, there's mutual oral. You are slightly more
restricted with positions for mutual oral, as you both need to be
able to reach each other's bits, but there are still a few to try.

69

This is the classic position for mutual oral, and for good reason.

The woman lies on her back. The man straddles her facing
her feet. Both bury their faces in their lover's bits.

Pros

It's an easy position to get into, and allows both partners
access to the perineum and anus.

Cons

The angle at which the penis enters the mouth can be tricky
and may result in teeth scraping across the penis. It's also
difficult to get deep penetration into the woman's mouth,
and can make her neck ache.

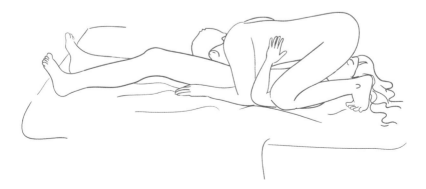

Reverse 69

This is the old classic, with a minor twist.

The man lies down and the woman straddles him, facing toward his feet.

Pros

The woman can control the pace as she grinds against the man's mouth. It's much easier for the woman to slide her lips to the base of the man's penis in this position than in the classic 69.

Cons

This can make the man's neck ache as he arches up to lick his partner. Some women find that tensing their thighs inhibits orgasm. There's a risk that the woman may smother the man.

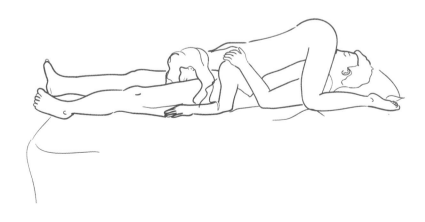

Doggie

This variation of reverse 69 requires more male thrusting but offers a different angle of approach to the penis.

   The woman gets onto all fours. The man lies underneath her with his head raised on pillows while the woman bobs her head down to suck his penis.

Pros

This offers the man a better view of the woman's breasts than reverse 69. It also lets him see her sucking his penis more clearly.

Cons

It can be hard on the woman's neck, and is trickier for the man to stimulate the woman's clitoris than in reverse 69.

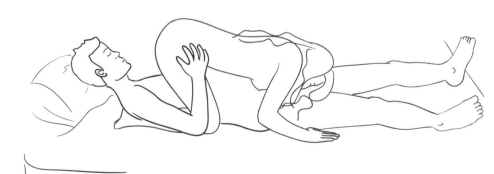

Troubleshooting

When you get cramp
Cramp can affect any sex session regardless of the position.
If you start to feel the burn, don't try to struggle on regardless.
Get out of whatever position you're in and stretch out the
cramping muscle. Your partner can always "keep momentum"
with a touch of self-pleasure. Once the pain eases, change into
another position and continue. If you suffer from cramps a lot,
see your doctor as it could indicate a mineral deficiency.

When you need to break wind
Don't think for a second that you can ease it out and your
partner won't notice. Tell them you really want to kiss them
to remove them from the "danger zone," then escape to the
bathroom to let rip.

When you hate certain positions
Don't do them. Just tell your partner that a position does nothing
for you. Alternatively, agree to compromise—you'll do a position
your partner loves but you hate if they'll return the favor.

Dos and Don'ts

For him

1. If you're in a dominant position don't get so carried away that you make your partner gag.

2. Do ask your partner if there's any position that she finds it particularly easy to climax in. Generally, it's harder for women than men to orgasm so the right position can make a major difference.

3. Don't complain if a woman refuses any "rear entry" positions. Many women are paranoid about the way their butt looks so it could really put her off if you insist on being that close to it.

For her

1. Do use different positions to explore your man's perineum and balls. They're often ignored erogenous zones.

2. Don't assume your man is a sexist if he likes having you on your knees in front of him. It's a great position, and you

can always get him to return the favor by kneeling to
perform oral sex on you.

3. Do warn your man if you think that a certain position could
   lead to teeth getting in the way.

For both of you

1. Do experiment with different positions. You won't know
   what you enjoy unless you try it.
2. Don't insist on a particular position that your partner
   dislikes. It shows a lack of respect.
3. Do be understanding with your partner if they have to stop
   for a quick break. Oral sex can be hard work. You can
   always pleasure them while they recover.

INCREASING THE PACE

Once you're proficient in the basics, it's time to move up a gear or two by pulling a few tricks out the bag. Whether it's superlative soixante-neuf, major multiple orgasms, or the old classic of deep throat, you can be sure that making the extra effort will put a smile—or orgasmic grimace—on your partner's face.

5

Mutual oral

Once you've got your individual oral techniques mastered, and you're looking for some new things to try to keep your oral sessions steamy and make sure your lover keeps coming back for more, then moving on to mutual oral is worth a go. It's the ultimate experience in shared intimacy and can also lead to simultaneous orgasms if you both pay close attention to each other's responses.

There's no magic trick to mutual oral really: just use the same techniques as you would if you were purely administering oral, and experiment with some different positions. However, depending on the position that you choose, you may find that a pillow under the man's or woman's head can help avoid getting a cricked neck.

Some people find it hard to climax during mutual oral because it's too distracting to pay attention to your lover while being pleasured at the same time, and so too difficult to relax and enjoy yourself. If this is the case for you, but your partner loves your mutual oral sessions, agree to keep it as a part of your repertoire but make sure you get "finished off" solo once they have reached climax. Giving each other a back rub afterward can help ease any aching muscles too.

Deep throat

Ever since Linda Lovelace first hit the cinema screens in the porn classic *Deep Throat*, men everywhere have been hoping to meet a woman who can take every inch of them. Deep-throating is now featured in almost every adult movie, no longer requiring the original film's exceptionally dubious premise that the woman had a clitoris in her throat. While it's not something that you should be expected to do, or feel bad about avoiding if the idea makes you (literally) gag, it can be a great way to give your partner pleasure, and it's not as difficult as you might think, as long as you approach it the right way.

To start with, make sure that your throat is as straight as possible as this means there's more room for the man's penis to fit in. Lying back on the bed with your head over the side is a particularly good position, though, be warned, it may give you a head rush. If it does, take a break. Passing out is not recommended as part of your sex life.

Next, raise your soft palate. This is the bit at the back of your throat that triggers your gag reflex. To raise it, all you need to do is flare your nostrils. OK, this isn't a great seduction look but your man should be so grateful you're attempting deep throat that he really shouldn't make any negative comments.

Now, the man should slide slowly into your mouth. Put your hands on his hips if he pushes forward too rapidly to control the pace. Deep throat should be taken at your speed, not his. As your throat gets used to accommodating his penis, push him slowly forward, each time allowing yourself to get used to the extra length before continuing. Once this is comfortable, start moving your head up and down. Stop if your gag reflex starts to rise, and simply lick the tip.

When you feel your man nearing orgasm (or, better yet, he warns you) either take him as deep down your throat as you can or move so that his penis is in your mouth rather than throat. The latter is recommended if you're a first-time deep throater as the spurts of semen can trigger the gag reflex. Once he's climaxed, smile sweetly and ask for diamonds. You'll probably get them.

"One trick I learned is to aim a man's penis into the side of my cheek rather than down my throat if I start to gag. It still feels like he's getting deep penetration but doesn't make me want to throw up. I cover what I'm doing with my hair so he can't tell the difference."

LIZZY, 36

TIPS FOR HER FROM HIM
The top five reasons men love deep throat

1. It's a bit pornographic. In fact, it's incredibly, massively, ridiculously pornographic. And men love performing anything they've seen someone else do on a video.

2. It makes her look insatiable…almost as if his bits were so incredibly tasty and he were so amazingly desirable, she just couldn't resist putting the whole thing in.

3. It concentrates her attention on the base of his cock…which is a very underrated part of the appendage. Yes, most of the nerve endings may be concentrated at the tip, but prolonged stimulation of the other end has the effect of producing amazingly deep and shockingly intense orgasms.

4. It's one of the best exercises in trust ever invented. She's trusting him not to thrust. Meanwhile, he's trusting her not to use teeth, or gag, or choke, or worse. As you can imagine, it's quite a daunting experience for the first-timer.

5. It pulls off the trick of looking incredibly sexy, but is also a bit of a rest period for him. In other words, despite being extremely intense, it's quite hard to come from deep throat. And just as well, really.

Multiple orgasms for him and her

You might think that multiple orgasms are a thing of myth requiring seven hours of Tantric chanting and a higher connection with your partner than merely wanting them, but that's nonsense. With a bit of effort and a few tricks, multiple orgasms are within your reach.

Multiple orgasms are much easier for women. Once she's come the first time, the man simply needs to keep stimulating her, but rather than touching the clitoral tip which will be far too sensitive, he should move his attentions to the clitoral hood, G-spot, or anus if she likes anal play. With enough practice, this should result in multiple orgasms.

For a man, you need to involve the prostate. Once the man starts coming, slide your finger inside his anus (making sure that you use a lot of lubricant, and have short nails). Feel around until you get to the prostate, a few inches up, behind the bladder and shaped like a walnut. Rub it gently using no more pressure than you would on an eyeball. With enough stimulation, you should be able to cause a second orgasm, and maybe more. Do warn your man first though—anal play should never be inflicted on an unsuspecting partner.

Alternatively, men can simply squeeze the Kegel muscles (see below) as orgasm approaches to ward off ejaculation. You can still climax without fluid coming out. Once the non-ejaculatory orgasm has passed, resume oral sex until ejaculation occurs.

Oral sex and toys

Then, of course, there are toys. Using a G-spot vibrator inside a woman while licking her clitoris can be thrilling, as can using a clitoral toy while lapping at the vagina. You can also get toys that attach to the tongue and vibrate to enhance oral sex. These sort of toys can be replaced by a vibrating waterproof cock ring if you're on a tight budget.

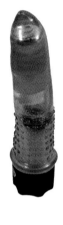

For men, holding a vibrator against your cheek while administering fellatio can add extra buzz, as can pressing a toy to the perineum. Just make sure that you use condoms on any toys that you share with your partner, or have separate toys of your own, to avoid any infections.

TRY THIS NOW!

Practicing your Kegel exercises will increase your chances of multiple orgasm. To do this, all you need to do is stop the flow of urine when you're peeing. This will identify the muscles you need to flex. Women can buy Kegel toners on the Internet—either weighted or sprung devices that are slipped into the vagina then squeezed with the relevant muscles. Men should drape a flannel over their erection then raise and lower it to increase the strength of their Kegels. This is best done alone unless you want to make your partner giggle.

Food play

Incorporating food into oral sex can spice things up. Strawberries and chocolate are obvious choices, but you could also try sherbert, champagne, and mint mouthwash which can all add an extra tingle to oral sex. Space Dust—the 1970s sweet that "burst" in your mouth can also feel thrilling when used on the genitals. However, any foreign substance can also irritate the delicate membranes of the genitals so make sure that you wash thoroughly if you engage in any kind of food play. Similarly, if you're smothering each other in cream, mousse, or any other substance before licking it off, make sure that you shower together afterward. Sugar left on the genitals can lead to yeast infections, and that's no fun at all.

Alternating a mouthful of warm coffee and semi-melted ice can also add an extra frisson to oral sex. However, make sure that the coffee isn't too hot, and never use non-melting ice as you could cause burns or ice burns. Basically, don't let your common sense go out the window just because you're feeling frisky and you won't go far wrong.

Female ejaculation

Many women worry if they ejaculate, fearing that they've wet themselves but in fact, the liquid released is prostatic fluid—the same stuff that's in male ejaculate but without the sperm. Not all women ejaculate, and the amount of liquid released in those that do can vary from a teaspoon to a pint, but it's certainly worth a try as some women say that it massively enhances their orgasm.

To start with, find the woman's G-spot. It's on the upper wall a few inches up, and will swell when rubbed. Do so in a "come here" finger motion. Stimulating the G-spot while administering oral sex can be an intense thrill. The woman may get an urge to urinate—this is normal as there's pressure on the bladder from G-spot stimulation, but the feeling should pass. Continue rubbing the G-spot and feeling it swell. If the woman bears down then eventually there's a good chance that she will squirt. You may want to practice this when not administering oral, and with a towel down, to start with, just so that you know how much liquid will squirt out.

Simultaneous orgasm

Although simultaneous orgasm seems the norm if you watch Hollywood films, in fact it's pretty rare. According to the Kinsey report, only 25 percent of men and 15 percent of women think that it's a "must," so the majority of people are more than happy to come separately.

Generally, it's the man who's likely to come first. As such, to increase your chances of simultaneous orgasm, the man should hold back for the woman until she starts to climax. During mutual orgasm, this can be helped by focusing on what he's doing to his partner rather than the sensations she's generating in him. As the woman starts to come, the man can return his attention to himself and/or think erotic thoughts to help trigger his orgasm. For some men, prostate stimulation can lead to immediate orgasm too.

Spending more time warming the woman up first also increases your chances of simultaneous orgasm. Spending lots of time on foreplay will both help ensure that the woman is closer to coming at the point at which you start. And don't just think that mutual orgasm is the man's responsibility. There's nothing to stop the woman from giving herself a helping hand to speed her climax: after all, she'll know exactly how and where to touch herself so she may as well use that knowledge.

The main thing to remember is that simultaneous orgasm is rare but practice makes perfect. And what a fun thing to have to practice . . .

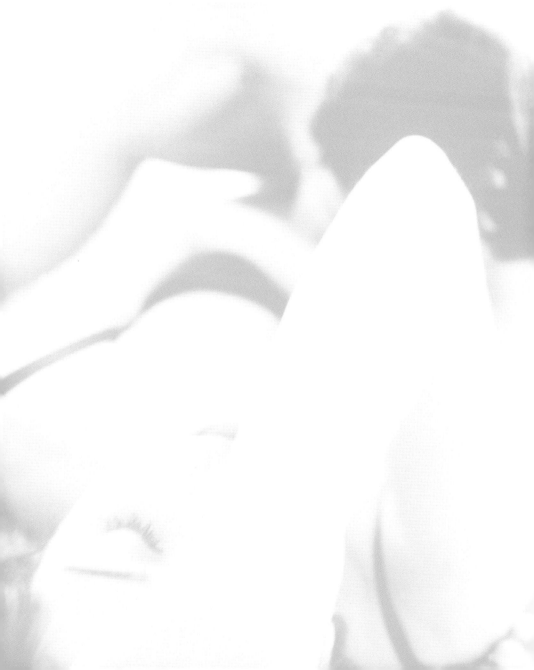

TIPS FOR HER FROM HIM
The allure of female ejaculation

Like 12-inch penises, massive plastic breasts, and five-female-one-male orgies, female ejaculation appears to be based firmly in the imaginary, overblown world of porn and has little bearing on more normal sexual experiences, yes? Well, no, actually—it's a genuine biological response, and it happens to far more women then you'd think.

Myth or fact

Although scientists are still arguing over the figures, it is estimated that almost all women are capable of it, up to 60 percent of women have experienced it to some extent, and nearly 20 percent have done so in a forceful manner at some point. This argument has even—pardon the expression—spilled over into the public domain; in the UK, the BBFC (British Board of Film Classification) will neither confirm nor deny whether they believe it actually exists, claiming that every video they've seen containing female ejaculation is actually a convoluted method of sneaking watersports in through the back door.

The source

Female ejaculation has nothing to do with urine at all. There are solid scientific claims that it actually comes from the Skene's gland, a pinhole-sized doo-dad located near the opening of the vagina. Like all parts of human anatomy, you'll find the size of the opening of the Skene's gland varies from woman to woman, which is a determining factor between a mild ejaculation (i.e., a damp patch in the bed) and a strong one (i.e., a porn-strength gush), or even none at all. In other words, there's nothing wrong with you if you do ejaculate, and nothing wrong with you if you don't.

Proof of orgasm

Naturally (and this should go without saying, really), most men love the idea of female ejaculation. Firstly, because they've seen it in porn films and it looks rather fun, as long as it's not on their bedspread. Secondly, because they love seeing the human body do weird things, particularly when it's someone else's body. Thirdly, and most importantly, it's bona fide proof that a woman has had a genuine, actual non-faked orgasm. Yes, there are plenty of other signifiers—flushed skin across the chest, tight breathing, dilation of pupils etc, but men really like to see a genuine result for their labors (not to put pressure on any women to produce the kind of jet spray seen in car washes, obviously). And to be fair, it's nice to let a woman come in your mouth and face for a change.

Giving the heads up

Obviously, if you're one of the 20 percent of females who do ejaculate forcefully, it's best to let any new partners be made aware of your little party-piece before you get down to anything—partly so he's not going to need his fingernails gently prised from the ceiling in shock (the first time you see it is a bit of an experience, trust me), but mainly for your benefit—because when he finds out what you're capable of, he's going to want to pay an excessive amount of attention to you down there . . .

Troubleshooting

When food gets stuck where it shouldn't

The golden rule with food play is what goes up won't necessarily come down so avoid this problem by never sticking anything inside a vagina or anus unless it has a flared base or string on it—thus ruling out most foods. If you ignore this advice and get something stuck, try to remove it with fingers first or, if it's stuck where the sun doesn't shine and won't cause you pain, try defecating. If that doesn't work, get thee to the ER and prepare yourself for a red-faced explanation.

When you throw up during fellatio

The only way to handle this horror is with laughter (once you stop throwing up and have cleaned everything up). Don't feel guilty if you're the vomiter—chances are it was because the guy was thrusting over-enthusiastically. However, use it as a lesson: don't be greedy and try to take more than you're capable of swallowing, or push too deeply if you're the man. Vomit and sex are a bad combination.

When the woman squirts across the room

The first time you ejaculate can be a shock, and more so if it's copious. Don't be embarrassed—it's not urine. It's merely a compliment on your lover's oral skills.

Dos and Don'ts

Do

1. Practice your Kegel exercises. They're one of the best ways to enhance your sex life.
2. Experiment with different techniques. If you don't try new things, you're more likely to get stuck in a rut.
3. Take anything that goes wrong lightly. Laughter is the best way to deal with most sexual mishaps.

Don't

1. Feel guilty if you can't climax together. Simultaneous orgasm is rare.
2. Put anything in the anus unless it has a string attached or a flared base.
3. Feel intimidated at the idea of using sex toys. Over half of women own at least one toy, so they're common but not a replacement for a loving partner.

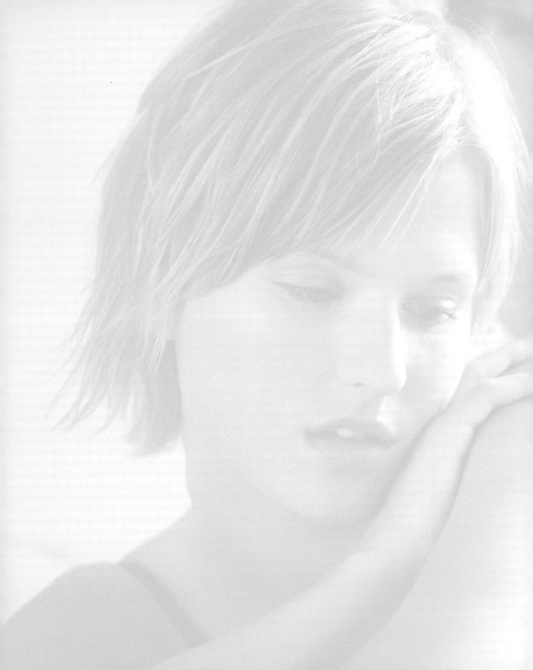

GOING WILD!

If you've read this far and practiced everything as you go along, by now you should be an oral aficionado. However, should you want to ramp things up a gear, there are a few kinkier twists that you can throw into the oral mix.

6

Analingus

Oral sex needn't just be confined to the vagina and penis. Analingus (aka "rimming") is something that many people find pleasurable and, as long as you follow the right safety precautions, it can be a sophisticated addition to your love life. Where oral sex was once a taboo, nowadays it's seen as a standard part of a healthy sex life. Analingus now fills the gap of being something a little bit forbidden, a little bit kinky, and, if done properly, a whole lot of fun. According to website queendom.com, 40 percent of men and 18 percent of women enjoy stimulating their partner's anus orally, and 69 percent of women and 77 percent of men enjoy having their anal region stimulated, so there are pretty good odds that it's something your partner will enjoy.

The big thing to bear in mind is safety. Unlike the genital region, you can still get infections from analingus even if you've both been tested for STDs and come out clean. No matter how clean you are, nasties such as E-coli can still lurk around the area so it's imperative that you use a dental dam. Viruses including intestinal parasites can lurk, waiting to give you fever, cramping, and diarrhoea, and if you ignore the dental dam advice you can also expose yourself to STDs including herpes, gonorrhea, HPV, and hepatitis. You may also be exposed to blood, and potentially HIV, if there are any cuts or tears in the anus. Similarly, if you move from anus to genitals without using a dam to protect yourselves, this can cause infection. To be on the safe side, use an alcohol mouthwash after rimming, as well as a dental dam during. Although there's no research that guarantees the effectiveness as a germ killer after rimming, at the very least it will also add a minty tingle to any further oral exploits. Don't think that merely washing thoroughly beforehand will protect you as bacteria can still linger.

Once you've got all the boring stuff out of the way, and have your latex dam in place, analingus is simply about exploring your partner's anus with your tongue. Try a number of different techniques to see which your partner most enjoys.

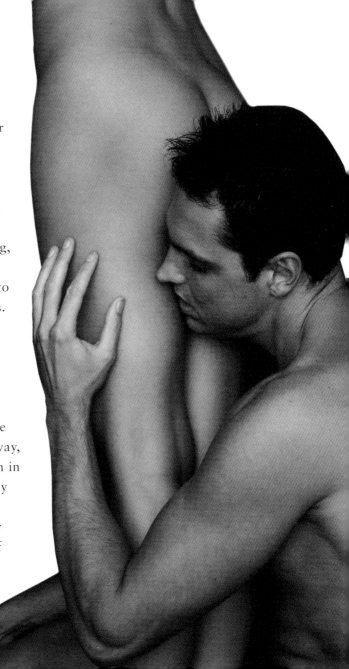

Techniques

You will need some analingus techniques to try on your partner, particularly if you are both new to the experience and looking to experiment. Practice these below to perfect your new oral skills.

Circling

Swirl your tongue around the entrance to the anus, gradually getting nearer and nearer the anus itself. This is a great move to start with as it helps relax the anus.

Dipping

Flicker a stiff tongue in and out of your partner's anus. Go slowly, getting deeper as your partner pushes back hard onto your face.

Perineal push

Press your tongue firmly against the perineum then draw it slowly back to the anus and either circle or dip your tongue around or inside the anus.

Sucking

Holding the dam firmly in place, suck very gently at your partner's anus.

Positions to try

As with oral sex, there are numerous positions you can try:

From behind

A classic position, though it does leave the "rimmed" partner in a very exposed position.

The receiver gets on all fours on the bed, leaving enough room behind them for their partner to kneel on all fours and easily access the anus.

Pros

This position provides access to the genitals as well as the anus, and it's easy to part the buttocks to improve access. It offers a graphic view which some men in particular may find a turn on. It's also ideal if you want to get toys involved.

Cons

Some people may find the position too animal or undignified to be able to relax, or that having their muscles tensed decreases chances of orgasm.

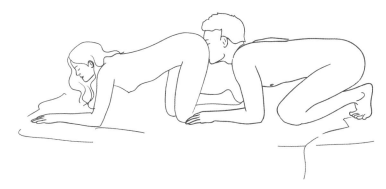

From above

This position can give the receiver a real dominant kick.

The giver lies back, facing upward, and the receiver straddles their body, leaning forward onto their elbows while the giver parts the buttocks with their hands.

Pros

This allows extremely easy access for the giver so is ideal for a first timer. However, it is a submissive position for the giver so they need to be comfortable with their sub side.

Cons

If the receiver gets carried away, it can be easy to block the giver's breathing. Leaning forward can become tiring for the receiver if they have to support a lot of their own weight.

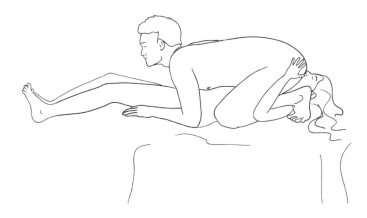

From the side

A lazy position for both of you.

The receiver lies on their side. The receiver lies behind them to lick their anal region.

Pros

This position allows both partner's easy access to the receivers buttocks making it easy to spread them for better access. It also lets both partner's lie down and relax.

Cons

If a partner is particularly large, the giver may get smothered by their buttocks. The giver doesn't have particularly easy access to other erogenous zones.

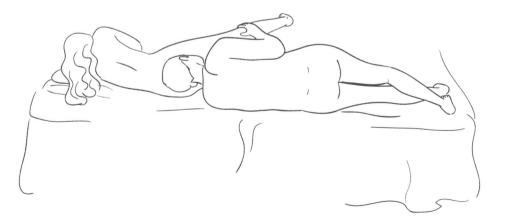

TIPS FOR HER FROM HIM
A man's view on analingus

Anal sex is no longer the strict preserve of gay men, or something that
only depraved hetero males wanted and even more depraved females
were willing to provide. And thank God for that; packed with sensitive
nerve endings capable of providing previously undiscovered sensations,
the anus is, for a lot of people, an erogenous zone that we're only now
becoming acquainted with, now that we're slowly casting off our shackles
of distaste for its primary, more prosaic function.

Experimenting

However, while a lot of us are au fait with the idea of penises, sex
toys, and digits probing around in that particular spot, we tend to draw
the line at rimming, for obvious reasons. Which is a bit strange. Although
it appears at first to be an incredibly extreme act absolutely sodden with
perversion and depravity, analingus could ironically be the key to the
kingdom for a vast amount of anal newcomers who want to experiment,
and the one act that can unlock the door and open up a whole new
realm of possibilities. Confused? Read on . . .

Small steps

Most men who haven't been initiated into anal play upon themselves
are at least vaguely aware that (gently) stimulating the prostate is a very
good thing, but are not very keen to try it out due to its association with
homosexuality. Analingus is the first step toward being coaxed into trying

it. No, we're not expecting your tongue to reach way up there, but when he's had some oral attention performed on the opening of his anus, he's going to be a lot more keen to try further experimentation. And it goes without saying that there is no greater bonding exercise than having someone swirl their tongue on that particular spot, because someone must really think a lot of you if they're happy to do that.

Reciprocating

Obviously, an act as personal and intimate as rimming cannot and should not go unreciprocated, and this is the other great thing about analingus for men; it can break down a lot of barriers when it comes to anal sex (which a lot of men would like more of, but refrain from initiating it because they assume their nice, innocent girlfriends would recoil in horror at the suggestion). There are just as many nerve-endings there in women as there are for men (come to think of it, it's the only true erogenous zone that both men and women possess), and they derive as much satisfaction from it as men do.

Easing into anal sex

Once they experience the sensations of a tongue in that particular area, women are generally more receptive to taking the next step toward anal sex. As a matter of fact, analingus is usually deployed as part of the steps to ward relaxing the anal muscles and making them ready for penetration. So there you have it; 50 percent kinkiness, 50 percent deeply personal and affectionate, a real gateway activity to a whole new world of sexual experience and a genuinely filthy thrill with a great view.

Outside the bedroom

If moving to different body parts isn't for you (or even if it is) you may decide to experiment with location instead. Oral sex outside the bedroom can be thrilling. Some people adore the exhibitionistic thrill of public oral sex. If you're one of them, it's worth practicing with discretion to avoid getting into trouble, and is easy enough to do if you follow a few guidelines. If you're not an exhibitionist and simply want to add a bit of variety, try the following:

Cunnilingus

- The woman lies back on the kitchen table and the man kneels between her legs.
- The woman sits on the washing machine on spin cycle while the man bends over her to administer oral.
- The woman sits at the dinner table and the man administers oral under the table.

Fellatio

- The man lies in a deckchair in the back garden "reading the paper" while the woman administers oral from the side.
- The man stands in the shower with the woman on her knees in front of him.
- The man stands at a solid balcony with the woman kneeling out of view fellating him.

Should you wish to take things further, do bear in mind that public sex is legally risky, and can result in imprisonment in some states and countries. As such, discretion is all important. For the least possible risk, the man should wear a long coat that can be used to hide the woman, and the woman should wear a short skirt and no underwear so that access is easy. Don't go for extended sessions—a quick and dirty fumble will be just as exciting and less risky. Take two picnic blankets, one for lying on and the other for rapid cover-up, or better yet, keep your oral sex excursion within the confines of your car. Pick somewhere that's quiet and well away from anywhere that children play. Make sure that the area isn't known for swinging in public either—unless you like the idea of other people getting involved. Other than that, just use whatever techniques work best for you both, and enjoy the frisson. Just don't blame me if you get caught—public oral sex is entirely at your own risk.

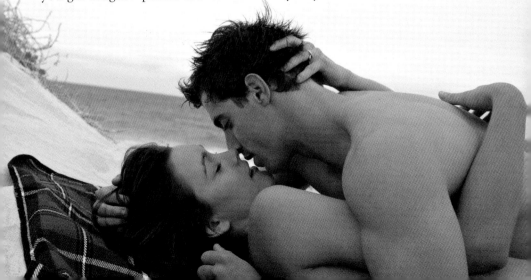

Sub/dom and oral sex

Then there's power play. Submission and domination are both popular kinks and adding a few tweaks to oral can help you become a sublime slave or decadent domme. Although it's entirely possible to have a wonderful oral sex session without any form of powerplay, the act does lend itself to master/mistress and slave scenarios. Adding any of the following moves to oral sex (consensually) will add a kinky twist. Do make sure that you've discussed your boundaries before you start playing, and agree on a "safe word" beforehand that you can use to stop proceedings at any point should you feel uncomfortable.

While you should never feel obliged to try any hardcore sex acts with a partner, experimenting with the milder end of the spectrum can add a whole new dimension to your sex life. Get creative too. As long as you ensure that you never restrict your partner's breathing, tie anything around their neck, or generally do anything life-threatening to them, whatever you experiment with in the confines of your own room is entirely up to you.

Dominant

- Pulling your partner's hair.
- Banning a partner from climaxing until you say so.
- Spitting in a partner's face.
- Slapping a partner's face (being careful to avoid the ear as otherwise you could break your partner's ear drum).
- Clamping your thighs around your partner's face.

Submissive

- Dressing in an outfit of your partner's choosing to perform oral sex.
- Being tied up while performing oral sex.
- Begging for semen or female ejaculate on your face.
- Performing deep throat until your partner decides to let you stop.
- Keeping semen/female fluids in your mouth after your partner has come until they tell you that you can swallow.

HIS AND HER ORAL SEX EXPERIENCES

"I think the best oral experience I ever had was when a guy at a party told me that he wanted to go down on me right there and then, and we did it in the bathroom. He never asked for anything in return, even when I offered. I've never felt so dominant in my life, and no, I never saw him again."

HELEN, 32

"The best blow job I ever received was from an ex who hardly did anything with her mouth at all. She pushed me back in a chair, took my cock out, and jerked me off very slowly while tracing the tip of my cock round and round her lips, with the odd drag of her tongue across the head whenever her arm got tired. She could do it for ages, but I could never last long enough to find out just how long, exactly."

CARL, 27

"If you can stand it, and it's been thoroughly washed out, a vibrating cock ring around the tongue does the business for my wife every time. And when you get used to the vibrations, it means I don't have to nosh away like a maniac and risk getting jaw ache."

BEN, 31

"My best oral moment was also my first time with an older woman, because she described every sensation as I was going down on her. It made me want to please her more, and making her come was ten times more important to me than the time I lost my virginity. I felt I had really achieved something, and I've never looked back."

JOHN, 36

"I wish it was as easy for him as it is for me, but outdoor spur-of-the-moment fellatio is a brilliant spontaneous trick. I've already done my boyfriend under a table at a party, in the park, and in a train bathroom—the novelty of it brings him off quickly every time. Shame I demand at least 20 minutes of attention, really."

KAREN, 26

"I was with my ex for five years. She loved the way that I gave her oral. After we split up, I played the field for a bit and didn't have any complaints, but when I met my new girlfriend she hated me going down on her. I thought she had some weird hang-up but one night after a few drinks she told me I was too rough with her. I was a bit hurt but I tried going down on her later that night and promised her that I'd be gentle. Instead of going into my usual routine, I tried different things and asked her to tell me what she liked best. It took a long time but eventually she came so hard that she cried! Now she asks me for oral all the time."

TIM, 32

Tips to try tonight

1. Offer your partner an oral sex session with no strings attached. Spend at least an hour exploring their body with your lips, fingers, and tongue and relish in the sensations and taste rather than waiting for them to return the favor.

2. Taste your own juices so that you know what your partner tastes when they go down on you.

3. Whisper sweet nothings into your partner's genitals while you go down on them. Even though they won't be able to hear you, the vibrations will enhance the experience.

4. Alternatively, get a vibrator and hold it against your cheek as you administer oral sex for even more buzz.

5. Make a fruit salad containing lots of strawberries and pineapple, and share it with your lover to make your juices taste sweeter.

6. Share a sexy shower together, making sure to get each other scrupulously clean. Massage each other's genitals with chocolate body butter after ward so that you taste extra sweet. Just make sure that it's cleaned off thoroughly if you

decide to have sex with condoms later as otherwise it may break the condom.

7. Think about the pubic hairstyle you'd most like your partner to have, then help them attain it. Once they've been suitably trimmed (or indeed, left au naturel) it's their turn to choose a pubic hair style for you.

8. Masturbate in front of your partner then let them lick and suck you while you continue to caress yourself. A joint effort makes for an easier orgasm.

9. Tell your partner three things that you love about the way that they go down on you.

10. Write a description of exactly how you'd most like to receive oral sex. Get your partner to do the same. Then swap papers and make each other's dreams come true.

When it comes down to it, great oral is about being willing to experiment and chalk any negatives down to experience. So grab your partner right now and get stuck in.

Index

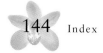

Picture Credits

Stefanie Coltra: pp. 83, 84, 85, 86, 87, 88, 89, 93, 94, 95, 96, 97, 98, 99, 129, 130, 131; Corbis: pp. 48, 64, 108; Dorling Kindersley Images: p. 127; iStock images: pp. 18, 115, 116, 117; Getty Images: pp. 2, 8, 11, 15, 22, 34, 39, 43, 52, 61, 66, 110, 125, 135, 140; Photolibrary: pp. 26, 56, 75, 80, 119;